METHODS IN MOLECULAR BIOLOGY

Series Editor
John M. Walker
School of Life and Medical Sciences
University of Hertfordshire
Hatfield, Hertfordshire, AL10 9AB, UK

For further volumes:
http://www.springer.com/series/7651

Population Epigenetics

Methods and Protocols

Edited by

Paul Haggarty

Rowett Institute of Nutrition and Health
University of Aberdeen
Aberdeen, Scotland, UK

Kristina Harrison

Rowett Institute of Nutrition and Health
University of Aberdeen
Aberdeen, Scotland, UK

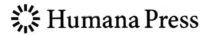

Editors
Paul Haggarty
Rowett Institute of Nutrition and Health
University of Aberdeen
Aberdeen, Scotland, UK

Kristina Harrison
Rowett Institute of Nutrition and Health
University of Aberdeen
Aberdeen, Scotland, UK

ISSN 1064-3745   ISSN 1940-6029   (electronic)
Methods in Molecular Biology
ISBN 978-1-4939-8333-9   ISBN 978-1-4939-6903-6   (eBook)
DOI 10.1007/978-1-4939-6903-6

This Humana Press imprint is published by Springer Nature
The registered company is Springer Science+Business Media LLC
The registered company address is: 233 Spring Street, New York, NY 10013, U.S.A.

Preface

Population epigenetics is an emerging field that seeks to exploit the latest insights in epigenetics to improve our understanding of the factors that influence health and longevity. Epigenetics is at the heart of a series of feedback loops that allow crosstalk between the genome and its environment. Epigenetic status is influenced by a range of environmental exposures including diet and nutrition, lifestyle, social status, infertility and its treatment, and even the emotional environment. Early life has been highlighted as a period of heightened sensitivity when the environment can have long-lasting epigenetic effects. Epigenetic status is also influenced by genotype at the level of both the local DNA sequence being epigenetically marked and the genes coding for the factors controlling epigenetic processes.

The promise of epigenetics is that, unlike the genetic determinants of health, it is modifiable and potentially reversible. The field of population epigenetics is of increasing interest to policy makers searching for explanations for complex epidemiological observations and conceptual models on which to base interventions. In order to fully exploit the potential of this exciting new field, we need to better understand the environmental and genetic programming of epigenetic states, the persistence of these marks in time, and their effect on biological function and health in current and future generations. This volume describes laboratory methodologies that can help researchers achieve these goals.

The most commonly studied epigenetic phenomenon in the field of population epigenetics is DNA methylation. Because of this, and the ready availability of methods to measure it, DNA methylation is probably the mechanism most amenable to study in population epigenetics in the near future. DNA methylation can be investigated at the level of individual methylation sites, specific genes, regions of the genome, or functional groups (e.g., promoters). An increasing number of human studies use array-based technologies to measure a great many methylation sites in a single sample. The trend is toward larger arrays measuring more and more methylation sites, but these tend to focus on the coding regions of the human genome. A significant component of the global methylation signature (average level of methylation across the entire genome) is accounted for by repeat elements. There are a number of classes of transposons and these include the long interspersed nuclear elements (LINE1), short interspersed transposable nuclear elements (SINE), and the *Alu* family of *SINE* elements. Approximately 45% of the human genome is made up of repeat elements, some of which are able to move around the genome and have the potential to cause abnormal function and disease if inserted into areas of the genome where the sequence is important for function. These are often heavily methylated, and this has the effect of repressing transposition and protecting the early embryo in particular from potentially damaging genome rearrangement during critical periods of development. Transposable elements are frequently found in or near genes, and the chromatin conformation at retrotransposons may spread and influence the transcription of nearby genes. There are particular problems in measuring this class of epigenetic regulators, and *Ha et al.* present a targeted high-throughput sequencing protocol for determination of the location of mobile elements within the genome. *Hoad and Harrison* consider the design and optimization of DNA methylation pyrosequencing assays targeting region-specific repeat elements. *Hay et al.* also focus on the noncoding genome where they describe online data mining of existing databases to identify functional regions of the genome affected by epigenetic modification and how these modifications might interact with polymorphic variation.

Chromatin is organized into accessible regions of euchromatin and poorly accessible regions of heterochromatin, and epigenetic control is fundamental to the transition between these states. Initiatives such as the ENCODE project have highlighted the importance of long-range epigenetic interactions to the function and regulation of the genome, and there is increasing interest in studying the large-scale epigenetic regulation of the genome in population studies. The chromosome conformation capture technique provides a way of assessing chromatin states in population studies. *Rudan and colleagues* describe the use of Hi-C while *Ea et al.* set out a quantitative 3C (3C-qPCR) protocol for improved quantitative analyses of intrachromosomal contacts. These authors also describe an algorithm for data normalization which allows more accurate comparisons between contact profiles.

The methylation state of the genome is a function of DNA methylation and demethylation, and much more is known about the former than the latter but that is beginning to change with our emerging understanding of the role of the 10–11 translocation (TET) proteins. *Thomson et al.* consider the potential functional role of 5-hydroxymethylcytosine (5hmC) and describe approaches to map this important modification.

One of the most important practical problems in population epigenetics results from tissue differences in epigenetic states. In many human cohort studies typically only peripheral blood or buccal cell DNA may be available but it cannot be assumed that epigenetic status in DNA from these sources reflects that in other tissues. The rationale for blood and buccal cell sampling is that epigenetic status within these cells is either indicative of key epigenetic events in the tissues and organs of interest or that it is simply a useful biomarker. However, this may not always be valid and heterogeneity of cell types, even within a blood sample, has the potential to confound research findings in population epigenetic studies. *Jones et al.* describe the use of a regression method to adjust for cell-type composition in DNA methylation data generated by methylation arrays, pyrosequencing or genome-wide bisulfite sequencing data. *Zou* describes a computational method (FaST-LMM-EWASher) which automatically corrects for cell-type composition without needing explicit prior knowledge of this.

In population studies there may be a limitation on the type and amount of material available for epigenetic analysis. *Butcher and Beck* describe nano-MeDIP-seq, a technique which allows methylome analysis using nanogram quantities of starting material. Most epigenetic studies are carried out in DNA derived from cells, but there is increasing interest in the potential for measurement of cell-free DNA in blood and other body fluids. *Jung et al.* describe methods for DNA methylation analysis of cell-free circulating DNA. Formalin-fixed, paraffin-embedded (FFPE) tissue is often studied in clinical research, but such samples are increasingly used in epidemiological study designs. *Jung et al.* also describe methods for epigenetic analysis of FFPE tissues and protocols for the preparation, bisulfite conversion, and DNA clean-up, for a wide range of tissue types.

The process of imprinting is particularly relevant to life course studies and the long-term effects on health of early environmental exposures. Imprinted genes are epigenetically regulated by methylation according to parental origin. The imprints are established early in development and, once set, the imprint persists in multiple tissue types over decades. There is evidence that some imprinting methylation in humans may be influenced by the early life environment. The characteristics of the imprinted genes—sensitivity to early life environment, stability in multiple tissues once set—make them particularly relevant to the study of early epigenetic programming of later health. *Skaar and Jirtle* describe methods for examining epigenetic regulation within regulatory DNA sequences with allele-specific methylation and monoallelic expression of opposite alleles in a parent-of-origin-specific manner.

Population epigenetics produces particular bioinformatic and statistical challenges when carrying out analysis of epigenetic data. *Horgan and Chua* describe methods for checking and cleaning data, the importance of batch effects, correction for multiple comparisons and false discovery rates, and the use of multivariate methods such as principal component analysis. In population epigenetics a further challenge lies in relating epigenetic data to phenotypic and exposure data in individuals and groups. Depending on the study design, epigenetic states can be considered as either an outcome or an explanatory variable and these authors describe how to match the statistical modeling approaches to the experimental question.

Our hope is that the methods presented in this volume will allow population researchers to exploit the latest insights into epigenetics to improve our understanding of the factors that influence human health and longevity.

Aberdeen, Scotland, UK   *Paul Haggarty*
                                                Kristina Harrison

Contents

Contributors

STEPHAN BECK • *UCL Cancer Institute, University College London, London, UK*

LEE M. BUTCHER • *UCL Cancer Institute, University College London, London, UK*

SOK-PENG CHUA • *Biomathematics and Statistics, University of Aberdeen, Aberdeen, UK*

FRANCK COURT • *Institut de Génétique Moléculaire de Montpellier, UMR5535, CNRS, Université de Montpellier, Montpellier, Cedex 5, France; Inserm UMR1103, CNRS UMR6293, F-63001 Clermont-Ferrand, France and Clermont Universite, Université d'Auvergne, Laboratoire GReD, Clermont-Ferrand, France*

PHILIP COWIE • *Institute of Medical Sciences, School of Medical Sciences, University of Aberdeen, Aberdeen, UK*

DIMO DIETRICH • *Institute of Pathology, University Hospital Bonn (UKB), Bonn, Germany*

VUTHY EA • *Institut de Génétique Moléculaire de Montpellier, UMR5535, CNRS, Université de Montpellier, Montpellier, Cedex 5, France*

RACHEL D. EDGAR • *Department of Medical Genetics, Centre for Molecular Medicine and Therapeutics, Child and Family Research Institute, University of British Columbia, Vancouver, BC, Canada*

THIERRY FORNE • *Institut de Génétique Moléculaire de Montpellier, UMR5535, CNRS, Université de Montpellier, Montpellier, Cedex 5, France*

HONGSEOK HA • *Department of Genetics, Rutgers, the State University of New Jersey, Piscataway, NJ, USA; Human Genetic Institute of New Jersey, Rutgers, the State University of New Jersey, Piscataway, NJ, USA*

SUZANA HADJUR • *Research Department of Cancer Biology, Cancer Institute, University College London, London, UK*

KRISTINA HARRISON • *Natural Products Group, Rowett Institute of Nutrition and Health, University of Aberdeen, Aberdeen, Scotland, UK*

ELIZABETH A. HAY • *Institute of Medical Sciences, School of Medical Sciences, University of Aberdeen, Aberdeen, UK*

GWEN HOAD • *Lifelong Health Group, Rowett Institute of Nutrition and Health, University of Aberdeen, Aberdeen, Scotland, UK*

GRAHAM W. HORGAN • *Biomathematics and Statistics, University of Aberdeen, Aberdeen, UK*

SUMAIYA A. ISLAM • *Department of Medical Genetics, Centre for Molecular Medicine and Therapeutics, Child and Family Research Institute, University of British Columbia, Vancouver, BC, Canada*

RANDY L. JIRTLE • *Department of Oncology, McArdle Laboratory for Cancer Research, University of Wisconsin-Madison, Madison, WI, USA; Department of Sport and Exercise Sciences, Institute of Sport and Physical Activity Research (ISPAR), University of Bedfordshire, Bedford, Bedfordshire, UK*

MEAGHAN J. JONES • *Department of Medical Genetics, Centre for Molecular Medicine and Therapeutics, Child and Family Research Institute, University of British Columbia, Vancouver, BC, Canada*

MARIA JUNG • *Institute of Pathology, University Hospital Bonn (UKB), Bonn, Germany*

MICHAEL S. KOBOR • *Department of Medical Genetics, Centre for Molecular Medicine and Therapeutics, Child and Family Research Institute, University of British Columbia, Vancouver, BC, Canada*

GLEN KRISTIANSEN • *Institute of Pathology, University Hospital Bonn (UKB), Bonn, Germany*

ALASDAIR MACKENZIE • *Institute of Medical Sciences, School of Medical Sciences, University of Aberdeen, Aberdeen, UK*

RICHARD R. MEEHAN • *MRC Human Genetics Unit, Institute of Genetics and Molecular Medicine, The University of Edinburgh, Edinburgh, UK*

COLM E. NESTOR • *The Centre for Individualized Medication, Linköping University Hospital, Linköping University, Linköping, Sweden*

MATTEO VIETRI RUDAN • *Research Department of Cancer Biology, Cancer Institute, University College London, London, UK*

TOM SEXTON • *Institute of Genetics and Molecular and Cellular Biology, CNRS UMR7104/INSERM U964, Illkirch, France; University of Strasbourg, Illkirch, France*

DAVID A. SKAAR • *Department of Biological Sciences, North Carolina State University, Raleigh, NC, USA*

JOHN P. THOMSON • *MRC Human Genetics Unit, Institute of Genetics and Molecular Medicine, The University of Edinburgh, Edinburgh, UK*

BARBARA UHL • *Institute of Pathology, University Hospital Bonn (UKB), Bonn, Germany*

NAN WANG • *Department of Genetics, Rutgers, the State University of New Jersey, Piscataway, NJ, USA; Human Genetic Institute of New Jersey, Rutgers, the State University of New Jersey, Piscataway, NJ, USA*

JINCHUAN XING • *Department of Genetics, Rutgers, the State University of New Jersey, Piscataway, NJ, USA; Human Genetic Institute of New Jersey, Rutgers, the State University of New Jersey, Piscataway, NJ, USA*

JAMES Y. ZOU • *School of Engineering and Applied Sciences, Harvard University, Cambridge, MA, USA*

Methods in Molecular Biology (2017) 1589: 1–15
DOI 10.1007/7651_2015_265
© Springer Science+Business Media New York 2015
Published online: 30 May 2016

Library Construction for High-Throughput Mobile Element Identification and Genotyping

Hongseok Ha, Nan Wang, and Jinchuan Xing

Abstract

Mobile genetic elements are discrete DNA elements that can move around and copy themselves in a genome. As a ubiquitous component of the genome, mobile elements contribute to both genetic and epigenetic variation. Therefore, it is important to determine the genome-wide distribution of mobile elements. Here we present a targeted high-throughput sequencing protocol called Mobile Element Scanning (ME-Scan) for genome-wide mobile element detection. We will describe oligonucleotides design, sequencing library construction, and computational analysis for the ME-Scan protocol.

Keywords: Mobile element, ME-Scan, High-throughput sequencing, Population diversity, Polymorphism

1 Introduction

Mobile elements (MEs) are a major component of the human genome. As a consequence of their transposition and accumulation, roughly two-thirds of the human genome comprises MEs [1]. Based on the transposition mechanism, MEs can be divided into two classes. Class I elements, also known as retrotransposons, use a "copy-and-paste" mechanism. During a process called retrotransposition, class I elements create new copies of themselves at different genomic locations via RNA intermediates. Class II elements, also known as DNA transposons, use a "cut-and-paste" mechanism and mobilize a DNA element from one genomic location to another. DNA transposons have been inactive over the past 30 million years in the primate lineage, while retrotransposons remain active in all primate genomes studied to date [2]. Retrotransposons are further subdivided into long terminal repeat (LTR) and non-LTR classes. Long interspersed element-1 (LINE-1, or L1) is a representative of non-LTR retrotransposon and encodes proteins necessary for autonomous retrotransposition [3]. Alu and SVA (SINE/variable number of tandem repeat (VNTR)/Alu) are non-autonomous elements that do not encode functional mobilization proteins by themselves. They rely on the enzymatic machinery of an L1 element to retrotranspose to other genomic locations [4–6].

MEs play a key role in genome evolution, creating structural variation both by generating new insertions and by promoting nonhomologous recombination [7, 8]. Mobile element insertions (MEIs) also shape gene regulatory networks by supplying and/or disrupting functional elements such as transcription factor binding sites, transcription enhancers, alternative splicing sites, nucleosome positioning signals, methylation signals, and chromatin boundaries [9, 10]. Some ME-derived or -targeted small RNAs, such as miR-NAs and piRNAs, also affect transcriptional regulation in the host genome [11, 12]. Therefore, it is important to determine the genomic locations of MEIs.

Because of their ability to transpose in the genome, MEs have also been used extensively in genome engineering. For example, transposon systems *sleeping beauty* and *piggyBac* have been used for mutagenesis and nonviral gene delivery [13, 14]. Once new transposons are integrated in the genome, it is necessary to determine their genomic locations. An efficient, high-throughput method is crucial to identify the insertion sites.

Before the high-throughput sequencing technology became available, transposon display methods were used to identify polymorphic MEI loci [15]. Transposon display methods identify the junction of an ME and its upstream or downstream flanking genomic sequence. Usually a primer specific to the ME of interest and either a random primer or a primer specific to a generic linker sequence are used to amplify the ME/genomic junction site. Once candidate MEI loci are identified, locus-specific PCRs are used to determine the MEI genotypes in individual samples (e.g., [16]). Recently, a number of efforts have been made to identify polymorphic MEIs using high-throughput sequencing technology (Reviewed in refs. [17, 18]). Although high-coverage whole genome sequencing is suitable for studying MEIs in different species, the cost is still too high for large-scale population-level studies. On the other hand, low coverage strategy such as the one adopted by the 1000 Genomes Project [19] is not ideal because it is likely to under-sample polymorphic MEIs. Mobile element scanning (ME-Scan) protocol adapts the transposon-display concept to the high-throughput sequencing platform and provides both high sensitivity and high specificity for MEI detection [20, 21]. Because the resulting sequencing library contains only DNA fragments at the MEI-genomic junction sites, it is a cost-effective way to identify MEIs for both large-scale genomic studies and transposon-based mutagenesis studies. Here we describe the ME-Scan protocol in detail. Although we use AluYb and L1HS family of MEs in human as examples to illustrate the ME-Scan application, the protocol can be easily modified for other MEs in other species by changing the ME-specific primers to the ME of interest.

2 Materials

2.1 Reagents

2.1.1 Oligonucleotides (Adaptors, Primers)

The adaptor and primer sequences used for human AluYb and L1HS ME-Scan protocol are shown in Table 1. To capture ME-specific fragments, two PCR amplification steps are required. Table 1 show oligonucleotides used for both PCRs. The first round ME-specific primers include 5′ biotinylation modification for bead capture and all primers include a phosphorothioate bond at the 3′ end for stability. In addition, current Illumina sequencing technology requires near random representation of all four nucleotides in the first three sequencing cycles to establish baseline signals and positions for base calls. Therefore, we incorporated three random bases within the second amplification primers.

For studies involving multiple samples, Illumina provides 6 bp index sequences for pooling multiple samples in one sequencing library. We tested 48 indexes and these index sequences have good uniformity and show no systematic biases. Therefore, we designed our customized linker sequences using the Illumina index sequences (Table 1).

2.1.2 Enzymes and Buffer Solutions

Several commercial kits were used in the protocol. For example, for sequencing library construction, we used KAPA Library Preparation Kit with SPRI solution for Illumina (KAPA Biosystems, Wilmington, MA, USA, cat. no KK8232). Other comparable reagents can be used as substitutes.

1. 1× TE buffer: 10 mM Tris (pH 8.0), 1 mM EDTA

2. KAPA Library Preparation Kit with SPRI solution for Illumina (KAPA Biosystems, cat. no KK8232)

3. Streptavidin-coupled Dynabeads magnetic beads (Life Technologies, Grand Island, NY, USA, cat. no 65305)

4. Agencourt AMPure XP beads (Beckman coulter, Indianapolis, IN, USA, cat. no A63880)

5. 2× B&W Buffer: 10 mM Tris–HCl (pH 7.5), 1 mM EDTA, 2 M NaCl

6. Agarose Gel: NuSieve GTG (Lonza, Cologne, Germany, cat. no 50084) and GeneMate LE (BioExpress, Kaysville, UT, USA, cat. no E-3120-500) (3:1)

7. 1× TBE buffer

8. 100 bp DNA ladder (New England Biolabs, Ipswich, MA, USA, cat. no N3231S)

9. Wizard SV Gel Clean-Up System (Promega, Madison, WI, USA, cat. no A9281)

Table 1
Oligonucleotides for ME-Scan protocol for human AluYb and L1HS MEs

Library	Description	Sequences (5′ → 3′)
L1HS L1HS L1HS	Biotinylated L1-specific primer cocktail for first amplification	/5Biosg/GGGAGATATACCTAATGCTAGATGACAC*A /5Biosg/GGGAGATATACCTAATGCTAGATGACAC*G /5Biosg/GGGAGATATACCTAATGCTAGATGACAA*G
L1HS	L1HS-specific primer for second amplification	AATGATACGGCGACCACCG1AGATCTACACTCTTTCCCTACACGACGCTCTTCCGATCTNNN GGGAGATATACCTAATGCTAGATGAC*A
AluYb	Biotinylated AluYb-specific primer for first amplification	/5Biosg/CAGGCCGGACTGCGGA*C
AluYb	AluYb-specific primer cocktail for second amplification	AATGATACGGCGACCACCGAGATCTACACTCTTTCCCTACACGACGCTCTTCCGATCTNNN AGTGCTGGGATTACAGGCGTG*A
Common	Typical Illumina adaptor pair including P7 region and individual index	CAAGCAGAAGACGGCATACGAGATCGTGATGTGACTGGAGTTCAGACGTGTGCTCTTCCGATC*T AGATCGGAAGAGCGTCGTG
Common	P7 adaptor-specific primer	CAAGCAGAAGACGGCATACGAGA*T

/5Biosg/: 5′ Biotin; *: 3′ Phosphorothioate bond
Underlined sequences indicate random sequences; *bold letters* indicate one example of Illumina index sequence

10. KAPA Library Quantification Kit for Illumina (KAPA Biosystems, cat. no KK4824)

11. Zero Blunt TOPO PCR Cloning Kit (Life Technologies, Grand Island, NY, USA, cat. no K270020).

2.2 Equipment

1. Heat block (Corning, Corning, NY, USA)

2. Covaris system with Crimp-Cap Micro-Tube (Covaris, Woburn, MA, USA)

3. NanoDrop spectrophotometer (Thermo Fisher Scientific, Waltham, MA, USA)

4. Magnetic stand (Promega, Madison, WI, USA, cat. no Z5342) or 96 well micro plate magnetic separation rack (New England Biolabs, cat. no S1511S)

5. Vortex mixer (Scientific Industries, Bohemia, NY, USA)

6. Thermal cycler PCR machine (Bio-Rad Laboratories, Hercules, CA, USA)

7. Gel electrophoresis system (Bio-Rad Laboratories)

8. Real-time PCR machine (Bio-Rad Laboratories)

9. High-throughput sequencer (Hiseq 2500, Miseq (Illumina, San Diego, CA, USA) and PACBIO RS (Pacific Biosciences, Menlo Park, CA, USA) were tested)

10. Water bath (Precision/Thermo Fisher Scientific, Waltham, MA, USA)

3 Methods

Procedures of the ME-Scan protocol are illustrated in Fig. 1. First, genomic DNA is randomly fragmented to ~1 kb in size (Fig. 1a). The DNA fragments are then end-repaired (Fig. 1b), A-tailed (Fig. 1c), and ligated to adaptors on both ends (Fig. 1d). DNA fragments containing ME-genomic junction are then amplified from the whole-genome library using ME-specific PCR (Fig. 1e). The amplified, biotinylated DNA fragments are enriched by streptavidin beads (Fig. 1f) and further amplified (Fig. 1g) into the final sequencing library. After the quality assessment (Fig. 1h), the library is sequenced (Fig. 1i). Below we describe each step in detail.

3.1 Preparation of Double-Strand DNA Adaptor

1. Mix equal volumes of paired oligonucleotides (100 μM). A pair of typical Illumina adaptors is shown in Table 1.

2. Incubate in a heat block for 5 min at 95 °C.

3. With tubes still in the heat block, turn off the heat block and allow tubes to cool to room temperature.

4. Store at 4 °C.

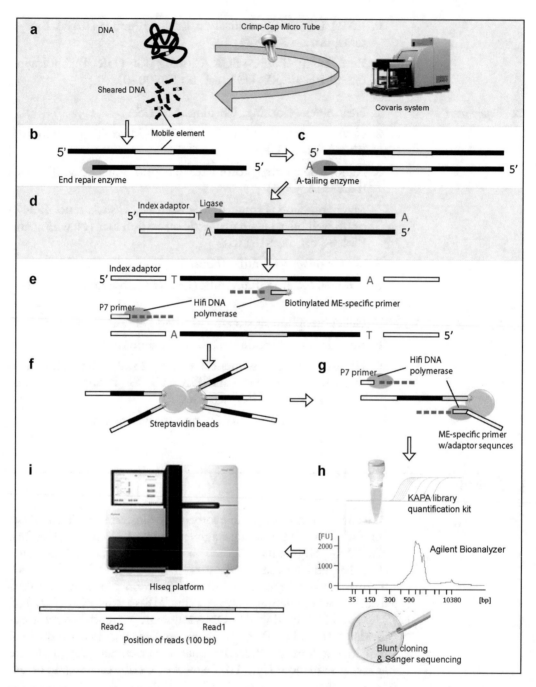

Fig. 1 ME-Scan library construction procedure. (**a**) DNA fragmentation; (**b**) end repair; (**c**) A-tailing; (**d**) adaptor ligation; (**e**) first PCR amplification; (**f**) beads capture; (**g**) second PCR amplification; (**h**) library validation; (**i**) high-throughput sequencing

3.2 Genomic DNA Fragmentation

1. Prepare 1–10 μg genomic DNA in 120 μL TE buffer.

2. Targeted fragment length is around 1,000 bp, and the operating conditions for the Covaris system are: Duty Cycle—5 %, Intensity—3, Cycle per Burst—200, Time—15 s.

3.3 ME-Scan Library Construction

3.3.1 Concentrate DNA Samples

1. Ensure that the AMPure XP Beads are equilibrated to room temperature, and thoroughly resuspended.

2. Mix 120 μl DNA fragments in TE buffer and 120 μl AMPure XP Beads per tube/well. For small sample size, mix in tubes; for large sample size, mix in 96-well plates. Because the total volume is more than 200 μl, use a microtiter plate (250 μl working volume) instead of a standard PCR plate for this step.

3. Mix thoroughly on a vortex mixer or by pipetting up and down at least ten times.

4. Incubate at room temperature for 5 min to allow DNA to bind to the beads.

5. Capture the beads by placing the tube/microtiter plate on an appropriate magnetic stand at room temperature for 10 min or until the liquid is completely clear.

6. If working with the microtiter plate, carefully remove and discard 120 μl supernatant (half of the total volume) per well. Do not disturb or discard any of the beads. If working with the tube, go directly to step 9.

7. Remove the microtiter plate from the magnetic stand, mix well and transfer the samples from the microtiter plate to a PCR plate (multichannel pipette can be used when processing multiple samples).

8. Capture the beads by placing the PCR plate on an appropriate magnetic stand at room temperature for 10 min or until the liquid is completely clear.

9. Carefully remove and discard the supernatant. Do not disturb or discard the beads. Some liquid may remain visible in the tube/well.

10. Remove the PCR plate from the magnetic stand, add 50 μl double-distilled water, and incubate at room temperature for 5–10 min to recover the DNA fragments.

3.3.2 End Repair Reaction

1. Assemble the end repair reaction in the PCR plate containing DNA fragments and AMPure XP Beads. For each well, add 20 μl End Repair Mix (8 μl water, 7 μl 10× KAPA End Repair Buffer, 5 μl KAPA End Repair Enzyme). For multiple library construction, master mix can be made for the End Repair Mix based on the number of libraries to improve the consistency. When making a master mix, add 1 or 2 more reaction volumes

to ensure sufficient volume. The same principle applies for making other master mixes in this protocol.

2. Mix each reaction thoroughly on a vortex mixer or by pipetting up and down, and incubate the plate at 20 °C for 30 min.

3.3.3   End Repair Cleanup

1. To each 70 µl end repair reaction, add 120 µl PEG/NaCl SPRI Solution.

2. Mix thoroughly by pipetting up and down multiple times and/ or by vortexing.

3. Incubate the plate at room temperature for 15 min, allowing the DNA to bind to the beads.

4. Place the plate on a magnetic stand at room temperature to capture the beads for 10 min or until the liquid is completely clear.

5. Remove and discard the supernatant.

6. While keeping the plate on the magnetic stand, add 200 µl of 80 % ethanol.

7. Incubate the plate at room temperature for 30 s to 1 min.

8. Remove and discard the ethanol.

9. Repeat the wash (steps 6–8).

10. Allow the beads to dry sufficiently for 5 min at room temperature and ensure that all the ethanol has evaporated.

3.3.4   A-Tailing Reaction

1. To each well containing the dried beads and end repaired DNA, add: 50 µl A-Tailing Master Mix (42 µl water, 5 µl 10× KAPA A-Tailing Master Buffer, 3 µl KAPA A-Tailing Enzyme).

2. Mix thoroughly by pipetting up and down multiple times, or by vortexing, to resuspend the beads.

3. Incubate the plate at 30 °C for 30 min.

3.3.5   A-Tailing Cleanup

1. To each well containing the 50 µl A-tailing reaction with beads, add 90 µl PEG/NaCl SPRI Solution.

2. Capture beads and perform cleanup as described in Section 3.3.3.

3. Remove the PCR plate from the magnetic stand, add 32 µl double-distilled water and incubate at room temperature for 5–10 min to recover the DNA fragments.

3.3.6   Calculate the Amount of Pre-annealed Adaptor Needed for Each Sample

1. Quantify the DNA concentration with 2 µl of each sample using the NanoDrop (As a quality control, the 260/280 ratio should be >2).

2. In ligation reactions, the molarity of sample (M_s) can be calculated using the following equation:

$$M_{s} = \frac{\text{Sample concentration}(\text{ng}/\mu l) \times 1,000,000 \times 10\ \mu l}{1000\ \text{bp} \times 650\ \text{Da} \times 50\ \mu l}$$

Then, the volume (in μl) of adaptor (10 μM) used in ligation should be:

$$\text{Volum of adaptor } (\mu l) = \frac{M_{s} \times 10 \times 50\ \mu l}{10\ \mu M \times 1000}$$

3.3.7 Adaptor Ligation Reaction

1. To each well containing 30 μl A-tailed product, add 15 μl Ligation Master Mix (10 μl 5× KAPA Ligation Buffer, 5 μl KAPA T4 DNA Ligase, supplied by the library preparation kit) and 5 μl adaptor (use the volume of adaptor determined in Section 3.3.6 and water for the remaining volume).

2. Mix thoroughly to resuspend the beads.

3. Incubate the plate at 20 °C for 15 min.

3.3.8 Adapter Ligation Cleanup

1. To each 50 μl ligation reaction with beads, add 50 μl PEG/NaCl SPRI Solution.

2. Capture beads and perform cleanup as described in Section 3.3.3.

3. Remove the PCR plate from the magnetic stand, add 50 μl double-distilled water and incubate at room temperature for 5–10 min to recover the DNA fragments.

4. Place the plate on a magnetic stand to capture the beads until the liquid is clear. Transfer the supernatant containing ligation product to a new plate. Discard the beads.

3.3.9 First PCR Amplification

Measure DNA concentration of each individual sample using NanoDrop. Normalize the sample concentration based on the NanoDrop quantification result and pool up to 48 individual samples with different index sequences together in one single tube with equal amount.

1. Set up PCR reactions according to Table 2.

2. Perform PCR reactions using the following conditions: initial denaturation for 45 s at 98 °C followed by 5–10 cycles of 98 °C for 15 s, anneal at 65 °C for 30 s, extension at 72 °C for 30 s followed by a final extension at 72 °C for 1 min.

3.3.10 ME-Containing Fragments Pull Down by Streptavidin Beads

Preparation

1. Dilute 2× B&W Buffer to 1× B&W Buffer with distilled water.

2. Calculate the amount of beads required based on their binding capacity [1 mg (100 μl) Dynabeads magnetic beads binds 10 μg double-stranded DNA].

3. Prepare appropriate amount of Dynabeads magnetic beads following the manufacturer's instructions.

Table 2
Pre-mix for PCR reaction

Component	For first amplification		For second amplification	
	Working concentration	Volume	Working concentration	Volume
PCR grade water		As needed		17 μl
2× KAPA HiFi HS RM	1×	25 μl	1×	25 μl
Adapter primer (P7)	10 μM	2.5 μl	10 μM	2.5 μl
(Biotinylated-) ME-specific primer (refer Table 1)	10 μM	2.5 μl	10 μM	2.5 μl
DNA		As needed		3 μl[a]
Total		50 μl		50 μl

[a]The template DNA solution contains the DNA fragments captured on the streptavidin beads

Immobilization of Nucleic Acids

1. Resuspend beads in 30 μl 2× B&W Buffer.
2. To immobilize DNA fragments, add an equal volume of the biotinylated DNA in H_2O to dilute the NaCl concentration in the 2× B&W Buffer from 2 M to 1 M for optimal binding.
3. Incubate for 15 min at room temperature using gentle rotation. Incubation time depends on the nucleic acid length: DNA fragments up to 1 kb require 15 min.
4. Separate the biotinylated DNA coated beads with a magnetic stand for 2–3 min or until the liquid is clear. Remove supernatant using a pipette while the tube is on the magnetic stand.
5. While keeping the tube on the magnetic stand, add 30 μl 1× B&W Buffer.
6. Incubate the tube at room temperature for 30 s to 1 min.
7. Remove and discard the B&W Buffer.
8. Repeat steps 5–7 twice, for a total of three washes.
9. Remove the tube from the magnetic stand and resuspend beads in 24 μl double-distilled water.

3.3.11 Second PCR Amplification

1. Set up PCR reactions according to Table 2.
2. Perform PCR reactions using the following conditions: initial denaturation for 45 s at 98 °C followed by at most 25 cycles of 98 °C for 15 s, anneal at 65 °C for 30 s, extension at 72 °C for 30 s followed by a final extension at 72 °C for 1 min.

3.3.12 Size Selection and Gel Extraction

1. Prepare a 2 % agarose gel using 3 quarters of NuSieve GTG and 1 quarter of GeneMate LE agarose.
2. Run the gel at 100 V for 55 min.

Table 3
The size of different components of the DNA fragments in a completed ME-Scan library

Parts	Size	Remarks
Read2 indexed adaptor	65 bp	The size of an index is 6 bp.
Read1 adaptor	58 bp	
Random sequences	3 ~ 5 bp	At least 3 bp random sequences at the beginning of Read 1 are required by current Illumina sequencing technology.
ME fragment	e.g., 123 bp for L1HS	The region from the ME-specific primer to the boundary of an ME.
Variable region	Variable length	The experimenter should consider variable sized regions such as a poly(A) tail at the 3′ end of an ME.
Genomic Flanking region	>20 bp	The genomic region should be large enough (e.g., >20 bp) to ensure the resulted sequencing reads can be mapped to the reference genome with high confidence.

3. Based on comparison to a DNA ladder, cut out the gel slice of the required size and place the gel slice in a 1.5 ml microcentrifuge tube. The required library size depends on the ME of interest and the sequencing platform. Refer to Table 3 for a size calculation example.

4. Extract DNA fragments from the gel slice using Wizard SV Gel Clean-Up System (Promega) following the manufacturer instruction. Elute DNA in 30 µl of elution buffer.

3.4 Library Validation and Sequencing

3.4.1 Validation of ME-Scan Library

1. Using Agilent Bioanalyzer, or similar technology, confirm the size distribution of the completed library. An example of the library size calculation is shown in Table 3.

2. Quantify the concentration of DNA fragments that can be sequenced by quantitative PCR using sequencing-specific primers (e.g., KAPA Library Quantification Kit). In general, the library should have a concentration of 10 nM or higher.

3. To validate the sequencing library, clone the library using a blunt-end cloning kit (e.g., Zero Blunt TOPO PCR Cloning Kits). Sequence a number of colonies to validate the DNA fragments within the library. Examine the DNA fragments in the library to ensure the presence of the proper library structure (e.g., sequencing primer binding sites, index) and the targeted ME sequences. We suggest that at least 24 colonies should be sequenced when a new ME-specific primer is used.

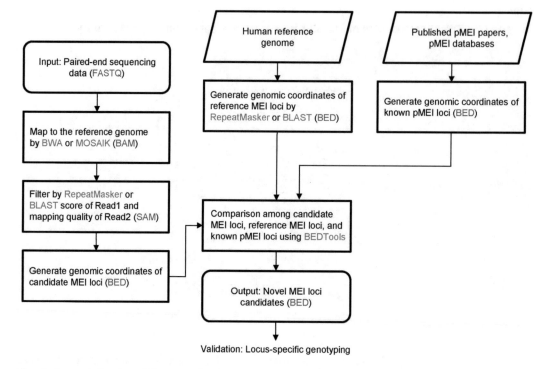

Fig. 2 Computational workflow for ME-Scan analysis. File format is shown in *red*, program name is shown in *blue*

3.4.2 High-Throughput Sequencing

Sequence the library on an Illumina HiSeq 2000/2500 platform using pair-end 100 base-pair format.

3.4.3 Analysis Pipeline

Figure 2 shows a flowchart of the analysis pipeline. First, raw sequencing reads were aligned to the reference genome using aligner such as BWA [22] or MOSAIK [23]. Pair-end reads that can be mapped to the genome were then filtered by two criteria: Read1 (containing targeted MEI sequence) is filtered using RepeatMasker [24] or BLAST [25] programs to ensure the presence of the expected MEI sequence; Read2 (genomic flanking sequences of MEIs) in each pair is filtered based on its mapping quality to ensure the unique mapping of the read-pair. Read pairs that failed either of the filters will be excluded from further analyses. After the filtering steps, the candidate loci are compared with known MEIs in the reference genome and known polymorphic MEI loci in previous studies and databases (e.g., [8, 19, 20, 26–31]) to identify novel polymorphic MEI loci.

4   Notes

1. When testing the protocol on a new type of ME, PCR-based locus-by-locus validation is strongly recommended to assess the sensitivity/specificity of the ME-specific primer.

2. Because PCR amplification is initiated from randomly sheared DNA fragments, a smear will be generated during the size selection step. Cutting a thin slice of gel (e.g., ~ 1 mm) can help to control the size distribution of the DNA fragments for downstream analysis. Also, the amount of DNA loaded for size selection should be carefully controlled. Overloading the gel could interfere with size separation of the DNA pool. Alternatively, if the size distribution of the final library is in a wide range, an additional size-selection step can be added after the first round PCR amplification (Section 3.3.9) to further improve specificity.

3. There are two types of bead-captures in the protocol for different purposes. Among the sections, different components (e.g., beads or the supernatant) were kept. The experimenter should pay close attention to these sections to make sure the correct component is kept.

4. We use the in-solution protocol from KAPA to improve the yield and reduce the cost for library construction [32]. In this protocol, AMPure XP Beads are kept in every step without replacement until the adaptor ligation step.

5. ME-specific primers should be reverse-complementary to a target region that is highly conserved in the ME consensus and close to the ME-genomic junction. If both ME's junctions (5'- or 3'-) are available, select the less variable junction is preferred (e.g., not attempting to capture the junction associated with the poly(A) tail at the 3' end of many MEs). Degenerate primers can be used if there are subtype mutations in targeted ME (refer to L1HS primers in Table 1 for an example). The ME-specific primer (non-biotinylated) for the second amplification can be designed in the internal region of the first amplicon (i.e., nested PCR) to improve the specificity of the protocol.

Acknowledgement

The authors declare no competing financial interests. We thank Drs. David Ray and Roy Platt for their valuable comments. This study was supported by grants from the National Institutes of Health (R00HG005846).

References

1. de Koning AP, Gu W, Castoe TA, Batzer MA, Pollock DD (2011) Repetitive elements may comprise over two-thirds of the human genome. PLoS Genet 7(12), e1002384. doi:10.1371/journal.pgen.1002384

2. Pace JK II, Feschotte C (2007) The evolutionary history of human DNA transposons: evidence for intense activity in the primate lineage. Genome Res 17(4):422–432. doi:10.1101/gr.5826307

3. Ostertag EM, Kazazian HH Jr (2001) Biology of mammalian L1 retrotransposons. Annu Rev Genet 35:501–538

4. Dewannieux M, Esnault C, Heidmann T (2003) LINE-mediated retrotransposition of marked Alu sequences. Nat Genet 35(1):41–48

5. Hancks DC, Goodier JL, Mandal PK, Cheung LE, Kazazian HH Jr (2011) Retrotransposition of marked SVA elements by human L1s in cultured cells. Hum Mol Genet 20 (17):3386–3400. doi:10.1093/hmg/ddr245

6. Raiz J, Damert A, Chira S, Held U, Klawitter S, Hamdorf M, Lower J, Stratling WH, Lower R, Schumann GG (2012) The non-autonomous retrotransposon SVA is trans-mobilized by the human LINE-1 protein machinery. Nucleic Acids Res 40(4):1666–1683. doi:10.1093/nar/gkr863

7. Burns KH, Boeke JD (2012) Human transposon tectonics. Cell 149(4):740–752. doi:10.1016/j.cell.2012.04.019

8. Xing J, Zhang Y, Han K, Salem AH, Sen SK, Huff CD, Zhou Q, Kirkness EF, Levy S, Batzer MA, Jorde LB (2009) Mobile elements create structural variation: analysis of a complete human genome. Genome Res 19 (9):1516–1526. doi:10.1101/gr.091827.109

9. Ichiyanagi K (2013) Epigenetic regulation of transcription and possible functions of mammalian short interspersed elements, SINEs. Genes Genet Syst 88(1):19–29

10. Cowley M, Oakey RJ (2013) Transposable elements re-wire and fine-tune the transcriptome. PLoS Genet 9(1), e1003234. doi:10.1371/journal.pgen.1003234

11. Piriyapongsa J, Marino-Ramirez L, Jordan IK (2007) Origin and evolution of human microRNAs from transposable elements. Genetics 176(2):1323–1337. doi:10.1534/genetics.107.072553

12. Rouget C, Papin C, Boureux A, Meunier AC, Franco B, Robine N, Lai EC, Pelisson A, Simonelig M (2010) Maternal mRNA deadenylation and decay by the piRNA pathway in the early Drosophila embryo. Nature 467(7319):1128–1132. doi:10.1038/nature09465

13. Wilson MH, Coates CJ, George AL Jr (2007) PiggyBac transposon-mediated gene transfer in human cells. Mol Ther 15(1):139–145. doi:10.1038/sj.mt.6300028

14. Mann MB, Jenkins NA, Copeland NG, Mann KM (2013) Sleeping Beauty mutagenesis: exploiting forward genetic screens for cancer gene discovery. Curr Opin Genet Dev 24:16–22. doi:10.1016/j.gde.2013.11.004

15. Van den Broeck D, Maes T, Sauer M, Zethof J, De Keukeleire P, D'Hauw M, Van Montagu M, Gerats T (1998) Transposon display identifies individual transposable elements in high copy number lines. Plant J 13(1):121–129. doi:10.1046/j.1365-313X.1998.00004.x

16. Xing J, Wang H, Han K, Ray DA, Huang CH, Chemnick LG, Stewart CB, Disotell TR, Ryder OA, Batzer MA (2005) A mobile element based phylogeny of Old World monkeys. Mol Phylogenet Evol 37(3):872–880. doi:10.1016/j.ympev.2005.04.015

17. Xing J, Witherspoon DJ, Jorde LB (2013) Mobile element biology: new possibilities with high-throughput sequencing. Trends Genet 29(5):280–289. doi:10.1016/j.tig.2012.12.002

18. Ray DA, Batzer MA (2011) Reading TE leaves: new approaches to the identification of transposable element insertions. Genome Res 21 (6):813–820. doi:10.1101/gr.110528.110

19. Stewart C, Kural D, Stromberg MP, Walker JA, Konkel MK, Stutz AM, Urban AE, Grubert F, Lam HY, Lee WP, Busby M, Indap AR, Garrison E, Huff C, Xing J, Snyder MP, Jorde LB, Batzer MA, Korbel JO, Marth GT, Genomes P (2011) A comprehensive map of mobile element insertion polymorphisms in humans. PLoS Genet 7(8), e1002236. doi:10.1371/journal.pgen.1002236

20. Witherspoon DJ, Xing J, Zhang Y, Watkins WS, Batzer MA, Jorde LB (2010) Mobile element scanning (ME-Scan) by targeted high-throughput sequencing. BMC Genomics 11:410. doi:10.1186/1471-2164-11-410

21. Witherspoon DJ, Zhang Y, Xing J, Watkins WS, Ha H, Batzer MA, Jorde LB (2013) Mobile element scanning (ME-Scan) identifies thousands of novel Alu insertions in diverse human populations. Genome Res 23 (7):1170–1181. doi:10.1101/gr.148973.112

22. Li H, Durbin R (2009) Fast and accurate short read alignment with Burrows-Wheeler transform. Bioinformatics 25(14):1754–1760. doi:10.1093/bioinformatics/btp324

23. Lee WP, Stromberg MP, Ward A, Stewart C, Garrison EP, Marth GT (2014) MOSAIK: a hash-based algorithm for accurate next-generation sequencing short-read mapping. PLoS One 9(3), e90581. doi:10.1371/journal.pone.0090581

24. Smit AF, Hubley R, Green P (1996-2010) RepeatMasker Open-3.0. http://www.repeatmasker.org.

25. Altschul SF, Gish W, Miller W, Myers EW, Lipman DJ (1990) Basic local alignment search tool. J Mol Biol 215(3):403–410

26. Ewing AD, Kazazian HH Jr (2010) High-throughput sequencing reveals extensive variation in human-specific L1 content in individual human genomes. Genome Res 20 (9):1262–1270. doi:10.1101/gr.106419.110

27. Iskow RC, McCabe MT, Mills RE, Torene S, Pittard WS, Neuwald AF, Van Meir EG, Vertino PM, Devine SE (2010) Natural mutagenesis of human genomes by endogenous retrotransposons. Cell 141(7):1253–1261. doi:10.1016/j.cell.2010.05.020

28. Beck CR, Collier P, Macfarlane C, Malig M, Kidd JM, Eichler EE, Badge RM, Moran JV (2010) LINE-1 retrotransposition activity in human genomes. Cell 141(7):1159–1170. doi:10.1016/j.cell.2010.05.021

29. Huang CR, Schneider AM, Lu Y, Niranjan T, Shen P, Robinson MA, Steranka JP, Valle D, Civin CI, Wang T, Wheelan SJ, Ji H, Boeke JD, Burns KH (2010) Mobile interspersed repeats are major structural variants in the human genome. Cell 141(7):1171–1182. doi:10.1016/j.cell.2010.05.026

30. Hormozdiari F, Hajirasouliha I, Dao P, Hach F, Yorukoglu D, Alkan C, Eichler EE, Sahinalp SC (2010) Next-generation VariationHunter: combinatorial algorithms for transposon insertion discovery. Bioinformatics 26(12):i350–i357. doi:10.1093/bioinformatics/btq216

31. Wang J, Song L, Grover D, Azrak S, Batzer MA, Liang P (2006) dbRIP: a highly integrated database of retrotransposon insertion polymorphisms in humans. Hum Mutat 27(4):323–329. doi:10.1002/humu.20307

32. Fisher S, Barry A, Abreu J, Minie B, Nolan J, Delorey TM, Young G, Fennell TJ, Allen A, Ambrogio L, Berlin AM, Blumenstiel B, Cibulskis K, Friedrich D, Johnson R, Juhn F, Reilly B, Shammas R, Stalker J, Sykes SM, Thompson J, Walsh J, Zimmer A, Zwirko Z, Gabriel S, Nicol R, Nusbaum C (2011) A scalable, fully automated process for construction of sequence-ready human exome targeted capture libraries. Genome Biol 12(1):R1. doi:10.1186/gb-2011-12-1-r1

Methods in Molecular Biology (2017) 1589: 17–27
DOI 10.1007/7651_2015_285
© Springer Science+Business Media New York 2015
Published online: 06 August 2016

The Design and Optimization of DNA Methylation Pyrosequencing Assays Targeting Region-Specific Repeat Elements

Gwen Hoad and Kristina Harrison

Abstract

Epigenetic modifications, such as DNA methylation, can contribute to gene regulation and chromosomal stability. There are several methods and techniques available for methylation analysis, ranging from global methylation to gene-specific targeted regions. Bisulfite conversion enables numerous methodologies to be used for downstream applications, including pyrosequencing which measures DNA methylation at an individual CpG site level. This allows specific regions of interest to be targeted for DNA methylation analysis. Designing and optimizing pyrosequencing assays correctly is vital for the interpretation of results.

Dysregulation of DNA methylation has been implicated in human diseases, with regions such as repeat elements commonly altered. Human population studies investigating these tend to use consensus sequences to target repeat elements. However, these elements have high mutational rates, particularly Alu sequences, which could lead to assay bias and masking of changes at a regional level. Therefore, it may be more beneficial to target specific repeat elements depending upon their chromosomal location, rather than analyzing overall methylation levels.

Keywords: DNA methylation, Epigenetics, Pyrosequencing, Bisulfite conversion, CpGs, Bisulfite sequencing

1 Introduction

The functional significance of DNA methylation, the most commonly studied epigenetic modification, can depend upon the location of CpG sites within the genome. These could range from CpGs at promoter regions at a particular gene of interest, to CpG sites at *cis*-regulatory regions. Human population studies tend to either examine global methylation levels or target gene-specific regions for analysis, and there are a variety of techniques to do this. The use of bisulfite converted DNA enables a range of downstream methodologies to be applied, both at a global and gene-specific scale. One of the most commonly used is pyrosequencing [1]. The bisulfite conversion enables non-methylated CpG sites to be distinguished from methylated CpGs.

Pyrosequencing is often referred to as the "gold standard" of DNA methylation analysis [2] and allows accurate quantitation at an individual CpG site resolution. After bisulfite conversion, PCR is used to amplify the region of interest and then a single-stranded DNA template is used for sequencing. This targeted technique enables analysis at gene-specific regions, with great accuracy. Pyrosequencing enables sequencing detection based on real-time pyrophosphate and subsequent fluorescence, which depends upon nucleotide incorporation [3].

Once a region to analyze has been selected for analysis, the assay should be designed appropriately. This process includes examination of the region to determine base pair location of CpG sites and the detection of any SNPs which may influence the accuracy of the assay. Optimisation of the designed primers is also required prior to analyzing cohort samples, including PCR mastermix components and cycle temperatures. To account for any potential bias that may arise from pyrosequencing batch analysis, controls should be run on each 96-well plate and sample layout should be considered accordingly.

Dysregulation of a number of regions, including repeat elements, have been implicated in human disease. Repeat elements account for ~55 % of the genome [4] with more recent studies suggesting that this figure could be over two-thirds of the genome [5]. Repeat elements are present within 25 % of promoter regions and thus the locational position could have a profound influence on transcription of proximal genes [6]. Short interspersed nuclear elements (SINEs) account for 11 % of the human genome with Alu sequences being the most common [6, 7]. Alu sequences are highly mutagenic with 213 subfamilies now identified, based upon sequence diversity and mutational events [8]. Targeting region-specific repeat elements could enable further DNA methylation information within a gene to be available and remove potential bias of analysis when using consensus sequences.

2 Materials

2.1 Online Resources

1. RepeatMasker: http://www.repeatmasker.org/.
2. PubMed: http://www.ncbi.nlm.nih.gov/pubmed.
3. Ensembl: http://www.ensembl.org/Homo_sapiens/Info/Index.
4. NCBI: http://blast.ncbi.nlm.nih.gov.

2.2 Samples Preparation

1. EDTA blood collection tubes.
2. QIAamp DNA Mini Blood QIAcube kit or equivalent.
3. PCR grade water.
4. QIAcube (Qiagen, Crawley, UK).
5. QIAgility robotic system (Qiagen, Crawley, UK).
6. SYBR® Green dye.

7. Rotorgene Q (Qiagen, Crawley, UK).

8. DNA standards.

2.3 Bisulfite Conversion

Commercially available bisulfite conversion kit.

2.4 PCR

Prepare all PCR solutions (primers and dNTPs) with PCR grade water. PCR reagents and primers were stored at −20 °C and all pyrosequencing reagents at 6–8 °C when not in use.

1. Hot Start Taq DNA polymerase.

2. PCR Buffer and $MgCl_2$ as supplied with Taq.

3. PCR Primers: 100 pmol/μL. Diluted with PCR grade water and stored in 50 μL stock aliquots. To prepare a working concentration of primer add 450 μL PCR grade water to a 50 μL aliquot of stock primer.

4. 10 mM dNTPs (deoxynucleotide triphosphates)

5. PCR grade water.

2.5 Agarose Gel

1. Agarose electrophoreses grade.

2. TAE buffer.

3. GelRed (Biotium, CA, USA).

4. 100 bp DNA ladder.

5. Loading Dye.

2.6 Cleanup of PCR Product

1. 70 % ethanol.

2. Milli-Q water 18.5 MΩ/cm^3.

3. PyroMark binding buffer (Qiagen, Netherlands).

4. Streptavidin Sepharose beads (GE Healthcare, UK).

5. PyroMark denaturation solution (Qiagen, Netherlands).

6. PyroMark wash buffer (Qiagen, Netherlands).

7. PyroMark annealing buffer (Qiagen, Netherlands).

8. Sequencing primer 10 pmol/μL.

2.7 Pyrosequencing

1. PyroMark Gold Q96 Reagents (Qiagen, Netherlands).

2. Milli-Q water 18.5 MΩ/cm^3.

3 Methods

3.1 Identifying Generic Region of Interest

1. Use PubMed and Ensembl databases to determine gene or region of interest. Gene name or chromosomal location (chromosome number and base pair location) can be entered into search filters.

2. Identify region of interest and take note of desired base pair location (*see* **Note 1**).

3. Within the PubMed database, click on FASTA tab.

4. Input base pair location to obtain relevant FASTA sequence.

3.2 For Identification of Region-Specific Repeat Elements

1. Search the RepeatMasker database for repeat elements within a gene, chromosomal region, or base pair location of interest.

2. Identify potential repeat elements for analysis, based upon position.

3. Use PubMed and Ensembl data to determine which identified regions to be targeted for further analysis.

3.3 Design of Pyrosequencing Assay

1. Export FASTA sequence of the desired target region into the PyroMark assay design software.

2. Select assay settings for PCR Primer and uncheck "allow primers over variable position." Select sequencing primer setting and uncheck the same box.

3. In the pull-down box select Methylation analysis (CpG) as analysis type.

4. Select the Graphic View Tab and from this screen, highlight the target region. Press start to generate primer sets (*see* **Note 2**).

5. If no primers are found on the upper strand, return to the original sequence editor and check the lower strand.

6. Once assay has been designed, paste the sequence for the whole PCR amplicon into BLAST on the NCBI website and search the SNP database (*see* **Note 3**).

3.4 Sample Preparation

1. Blood samples collected from participants using EDTA tubes and stored on ice.

2. Whole blood centrifuged at $1200 \times g$ for 15 min at 4 °C.

3. Plasma, buffy coat, and red blood cells separated and stored at −80 °C.

3.5 DNA Extraction and Quantification

1. 200 μL of buffy coat sample used as the starting material for DNA extraction (*see* **Note 4**).

2. QIAamp DNA Mini Blood QIAcube kit and a QIAcube used for DNA extraction.

3. Prepare samples for DNA quantification using a QIAgility robotic system.

4. Prepare a standard curve using DNA standards of concentrations 10, 5, 2.5, and 1.25 ng/μL.

5. Quantify DNA using SYBR® Green dye on a Rotorgene Q, following the manufactures protocol.

3.6 Bisulfite Conversion

1. Pipette DNA and water into a 96-well reaction plate, with a final volume of 40 μL, concentration of 12.5 ng/μL (*see* **Note 5**). Carry out conversion reaction and cleanup of DNA as per manufacturer's instructions for the bisulfite conversion kit in use.

2. At end of DNA cleanup process, add a volume of PCR grade water to each well of the plate to achieve a final concentration of 2 ng/μL DNA (assuming 100 % recovery of starting DNA).

3. Aliquot 10 μL of these DNA solutions into the required number of 96-well PCR reaction plates. Seal plates and store at −80 °C until required for further analyses (*see* **Note 6**).

3.7 PCR Optimisation

1. Defrost, vortex and spin PCR buffer, dNTP solution, forward and reverse primers, magnesium chloride and Q solution. Leave Taq polymerase in freezer until immediately before it is required. Do not vortex Taq, tap tube gently to mix then spin briefly.

2. Prepare control samples (*see* **Note 7**) for PCR optimisation.

3. Magnesium chloride concentrations (1.5 and 3 mM) and the addition of Q solution were trialled for PCR master mixes (*see* **Note 8**).

4. PCR optimisation carried out for each primer set (*see* **Note 9**).

3.8 Agarose Gel

1. Set up casting tray with combs and end stops in tank.

2. Weigh Agarose into a conical flask (0.6 g for a 2 % gel).

3. Add 30 mL 1× TAE buffer, cover with cling film and pierce.

4. Microwave on full power for about 40 s until agarose has dissolved.

5. Add 3 μL GelRed dye directly into the melted agarose and gently swirl flask.

6. Pour agarose solution into casting tray and leave to set (approx. 20 min).

7. Pipette 5 μL of PCR product from PCR optimisation and 1 μL of loading dye into 0.2 mL tubes or a 96-well plate. Also prepare 5 μL DNA ladder and 1 μL loading dye.

8. Remove combs and end stops from tank. Fill with 1× TAE buffer until gel is just covered.

9. Mix each sample by pipetting up and down and add 5 μL to each well.

10. Attach power pack and run at 80 mA for 20 min.

11. View gel in the transilluminator. Control samples with the clearest and most specific band should be selected as the optimized PCR conditions to use for sample analysis.

3.9 PCR of Samples

1. Defrost bisulfite converted DNA. Centrifuge 96-well plate briefly.

2. Prepare a master mix for required number of samples plus approx. 10 % to allow for losses during pipetting (for 96-well plates prepare enough for 104 samples).

   For one sample:

PCR buffer	2.5 μL
dNTP 10 mM	2.0 μL
Forward primer 10 pmol/μL	0.5 μL
Reverse primer 10 pmol/μL	0.5 μL
MgCl$_2$	Dependant on individual assay
Q solution	Dependant on individual assay
HotStarTaq	0.16 μL
Water	9.3 μL.[a]

[a]If MgCl$_2$ or Q solution used decrease volume of water by volume of MgCl$_2$ or Q solution.

3. Mix well and add 15 μL of master mix to each well of the 96-well plate. Seal the plate and centrifuge briefly.

4. Place the plate in the thermal cycler and run using the optimized cycling program.

5. At end of cycling process, store plate at 4 °C if processing within 24 h, otherwise store at −20 °C (*see* **Note 10**).

6. Set up an agarose gel check as detailed in Section 3.8.

7. Confirm that only one band visible for each sample and that it is the expected size of amplicon for that specific PCR reaction.

3.10 Cleanup of PCR Product

1. Remove all solutions from fridge and leave to reach room temperature.

2. Place thermoplate and cover on heating block set to 80 °C.

3. Fill troughs on vacuum prep station.
   - Trough 1: 70 % ethanol
   - Trough 2: Denaturation solution
   - Trough 3: Washing buffer
   - Trough 4: High purity water
   - Parking trough: High purity water

4. Transfer appropriate volume of PCR product to a 96-well plate (normally 5 or 10 μL); add water to bring total volume to 40 mL.

5. Shake bottle of Sepharose beads thoroughly until a homogenous solution obtained.

6. Prepare Binding Buffer/Streptavidin Sepharose bead mix. 38 μL Binding buffer and 2 μL beads are required per well. Prepare volume required for number of wells plus two extra volumes.

7. Mix thoroughly; add 40 μL to each well of plate.

8. Seal plate, place on shaker for a minimum of 10 min to disperse beads.

9. While plate is shaking prepare pyrosequencing plate. Mix together the required volumes of sequencing primer and annealing buffer: 0.36 μL sequencing primer (10 pmol/μL) and 11.64 μL annealing buffer per well.

10. Mix thoroughly and add 12 μL to each well of a PSQ HS 96 plate.

11. Place this plate in position on vacuum prep station (park position).

12. Switch on vacuum pump, open the vacuum switch (ON) check vacuum has been attained; needle on gauge should be beyond the red range. Wash the vac prep tool by placing it in park position and allow water to flush through probes for approx. 20 s. Remove prep tool from trough and allow water to drain from filter probes. Close vacuum switch and return prep tool to park position.

13. Remove plate containing beads and PCR product from shaker and remove film seal. Work quickly so that beads do not settle to bottom of wells. Capturing must take place within 3 min of removal from shaker.

14. Place plate on vac prep station. Check that well A1 is in correct position. Open the vacuum switch (ON). Capture the beads by *slowly* lowering the vac prep tool into the plate. Wait for all liquid to be aspirated from wells then check all beads have been captured onto probe tips.

15. Move the prep tool into ethanol and allow to flush through filters for 5 s.

16. Move to Denaturation buffer and allow to flush through filters for 5 s.

17. Move the prep tool to washing buffer and allow to flush through for 5 s.

18. Allow all liquid to drain from filter probes by raising the prep tool and holding it beyond 90° vertical. Hold for a few seconds until no further liquid being pulled through tubing.

19. *Close the vacuum* (switch in OFF position).

20. Lower probes into PSQ plate, probes should be resting on bottom of wells. Shake *vigorously* to release beads into annealing solution (*see* **Note 11**).

21. Move prep tool into trough 4 and agitate prep tool for 10 s. If preparing further plates can proceed as above protocol. If last plate then wash filter probes by placing prep tool in park position and flushing through with water for approx. 20 s. If there is 70 % ethanol remaining in trough can also give a final rinse with ethanol.

22. Place PSQ plate on thermoplate and cover with lid. Heat at 80 °C for 2 min (no longer than 3 min).

23. Allow plate to cool to room temperature then seal. Plate can be analyzed immediately or stored for several weeks in fridge (*see* **Note 12**). If plate is stored for any length of time then repeat heating step prior to analysis on Pyrosequencer.

24. Return all solutions to fridge. Empty and rinse troughs with deionised water. Empty and rinse vacuum prep station waste collection bottle.

3.11 Operation of Pyrosequencer

1. Switch on computer connected to pyrosequencer then switch on pyrosequencer. Allow 1 h for detector to warm up.

2. Prepare enzyme and substrate solutions according to information on pack.

3. Prepare a plate map containing sample ID using Excel.

4. Open CpG software, click on "New Run."

5. Copy and paste plate layout from prepared Excel file.

6. Go back to CpG software and right click on well A1, click "Paste Sample Layout."

7. Highlight wells for each assay. Go to Assay folder and click then drag appropriate assay to the wells.

8. Enter instrument parameters using pull-down menu.

9. Click on "Tools," "Volume Information."

10. Add stated volumes to appropriate dispensing tips. For nucleotide tips tap gently to ensure no air bubbles at base of tip. Ensure that tips are in the correct position.

11. Place tip holder into instrument. Open lid using icon in CpG software and insert dispensing test plate (*see* **Note 13**).

12. Close lid and click on icon for test dispense. Wait for test to occur, open lid and check that six drops are visible. If not try tapping tips to remove any bubbles and run test again. If still no drops then replace the appropriate tip with a new one.

13. If tip dispensation test successful, remove test plate from instrument (*see* **Note 14**).

14. Remove seal from PSQ plate and place plate in instrument, close lid using software.

15. Press run button (*see* **Note 15**).

16. At end of run press analyze and save data.

17. Remove plate (discard) and tip holder. Rinse reagent tips with high purity water then cover top with finger to force water through the tips. Rinse NDTs with high purity water taking care *not* to get water on end of tip (*see* **Note 16**). Place tips in storage box (*see* **Note 17**).

18. To switch off instrument the shutdown instrument command in the CpG software *MUST* be used. Power can then be switched off at instrument once computer states it is safe to do so.

4   Notes

1. Use Ensembl to identify CpG islands and ensure that selected region of interest does not contain a high number of genetic variations.

2. Ideally primer sets of a score between 80 and 100 should be selected, but often the best score obtained is much lower.

3. Identify where any SNPs are. If SNPs occur at CpG sites or within desired primers, a new assay will need to be designed. If SNPs occur within the sequence to analyze these will need to be accounted for when the sequence is entered into the Pyro-Q CpG software.

4. Buffy coat samples can yield 5–10 times more DNA than a similar volume of whole blood. Research into the heterogeneity of cell type composition should be considered when selecting which sample type to use for analysis. For regions such as repeat elements, cell type composition does not have a significant influence upon methylation level.

5. When assigning samples to the 96-well plate for a case control study always ensure there are equal numbers of cases and controls on each plate. Otherwise between-plate variation could lead to a bias in data obtained. Include on every plate at least two replicates of a quality control DNA sample. Analyses of data from this sample will indicate the level of between-plate variation.

6. Aliquoting the bisulfite converted DNA at this stage removes the risk of damaging the DNA by multiple thaw–freeze cycles. This bisulfite converted DNA should be stable for 36 months.

7. Control samples used for PCR optimisation were in-house bisulfite converted pooled DNA, utilized for all assay preparations.

8. Magnesium chloride concentration can reduce primer dimer risk and is a required cofactor for Taq polymerase. PCR buffer already contains a concentration of 1.5 mM. Q solution can aid in the amplification of GC-rich templates.

9. Ta (annealing temperature) is dependent on individual primers. Optimize each PCR primer set by trialling annealing temperatures, starting point taken as 5 °C below the melting temperature of the PCR primers.

10. To further reduce potential of batch effects, all PCR runs should be carried out on the same day using the same reagents, or as close together as possible. This decreases the risk of variability between PCR successes.

11. When shaking probes vigorously a mixture of rocking towards and away from you can used with shaking probe from the tube end ensures that all probes have been agitated to remove beads into the annealing/primer solution.

12. If analyzing PSQ plates within 24 h they can be left at room temperature (for example overnight) and then reheated at 80 °C prior to pyrosequencing. Analysis of plates tend to more successful (less "checks" or "failed" samples) than those which are stored in the fridge overnight then reheated.

13. When opening and closing lid of pyrosequencer the icons in the CpG software must also be used to open and close the plate holder. Do not open the outer lid of the pyrosequencer until a couple of seconds after the instrument has stopped making a noise (opening and closing plate holder) as this can lead to an error screen occurring and the CpG software shutting down.

14. Dispensing test plate comprises of a PSQ plate which has been sealed so that tips test will show if liquid has been dispensed from the six tips. If there are not six drops of liquid visible after test dispension, attempt again after ensuring there are no bubbles or blockages within any of the tips.

15. If doing more than one PSQ plate, store reagents (enzyme, substrate, and nucleotides) in the fridge between runs as this reduces the chance of tips blocking during runs.

16. If tips are to be used again within 24 h they can remain in the tip holder and be stored in the fridge, inside the black box. Ensure that there are some volumes of NDTs remaining within the tips prior to storage to minimize the risk of tips blocking upon reuse.

17. NDT tips are less likely to block if they are not washed but used again within 24 h of previous run.

References

1. Frommer M, McDonald LE, Millar DS, Collis CM, Watt F, Grigg GW, Molloy PL, Paul CL (1992) A genomic sequencing protocol that yields a positive display of 5-methylcytosine residues in individual DNA strands. Proc Natl Acad Sci 89(5):1827–1831

2. Clark SJ, Statham A, Stirzaker C, Molloy PL, Frommer M (2006) DNA methylation: bisulphite modification and analysis. Nat Protoc 1 (5):2353–2364

3. Ronaghi M, Uhlén M, Nyrén P (1998) A Sequencing Method Based on Real-Time Pyrophosphate. Science 281(5375):363–365

4. Lander ES, Linton LM, Birren B, Nusbaum C, Zody MC, Baldwin J, Devon K, Dewar K, Doyle M, FitzHugh W (2001) Initial sequencing and analysis of the human genome. Nature 409 (6822):860–921

5. de Koning AJ, Gu W, Castoe TA, Batzer MA, Pollock DD (2011) Repetitive elements may comprise over two-thirds of the human genome. PLoS Genet 7(12), e1002384

6. Cordaux R, Batzer MA (2009) The impact of retrotransposons on human genome evolution. Nat Rev Genet 10(10):691–703

7. Levin HL, Moran JV (2011) Dynamic interactions between transposable elements and their hosts. Nat Rev Genet 12(9):615–627

8. Liu GE, Alkan C, Jiang L, Zhao S, Eichler EE (2009) Comparative analysis of Alu repeats in primate genomes. Genome Res 19 (5):876–885

Methods in Molecular Biology (2017) 1589: 29–45
DOI 10.1007/7651_2015_263
© Springer Science+Business Media New York 2015
Published online: 30 May 2016

Determining Epigenetic Targets: A Beginner's Guide to Identifying Genome Functionality Through Database Analysis

Elizabeth A. Hay, Philip Cowie, and Alasdair MacKenzie

Abstract

There can now be little doubt that the cis-regulatory genome represents the largest information source within the human genome essential for health. In addition to containing up to five times more information than the coding genome, the cis-regulatory genome also acts as a major reservoir of disease-associated polymorphic variation. The cis-regulatory genome, which is comprised of enhancers, silencers, promoters, and insulators, also acts as a major functional target for epigenetic modification including DNA methylation and chromatin modifications. These epigenetic modifications impact the ability of cis-regulatory sequences to maintain tissue-specific and inducible expression of genes that preserve health. There has been limited ability to identify and characterize the functional components of this huge and largely misunderstood part of the human genome that, for decades, was ignored as "Junk" DNA. In an attempt to address this deficit, the current chapter will first describe methods of identifying and characterizing functional elements of the cis-regulatory genome at a genome-wide level using databases such as ENCODE, the UCSC browser, and NCBI. We will then explore the databases on the UCSC genome browser, which provides access to DNA methylation and chromatin modification datasets. Finally, we will describe how we can superimpose the huge volume of study data contained in the NCBI archives onto that contained within the UCSC browser in order to glean relevant in vivo study data for any locus within the genome. An ability to access and utilize these information sources will become essential to informing the future design of experiments and subsequent determination of the role of epigenetics in health and disease and will form a critical step in our development of personalized medicine.

Keywords: Cis-regulatory genome, Polymorphic variation, Epigenetics, DNA methylation, Chromatin modification, Genome databases, Bioinformatics

1 Introduction

Epigenetics is the term used to define heritable changes to the genome that result in changes to gene expression but which do not involve changes in the underlying DNA sequences [1]. The molecular mechanisms of epigenetics include DNA methylation, posttranscriptional histone modification, and ATP-dependent chromatin remodeling [1]. Environmental influences such as stress and nutrition, as well as aging, are thought to be major contributors to epigenetic alterations of the genome and have an important effect on an individual's health, as well as susceptibility, to a wide variety of diseases.

The current chapter represents a "beginner's guide" to identifying functional targets for epigenetic modification within the human noncoding genome, using freely available online repositories of genomic data. It is not our intention to describe these databases in major detail. Instead it is hoped that by introducing these databases and guiding the reader through the initial steps of accessing the data, we can bridge the perceived gap between the biomedical scientist interested in the effects of epigenetic modification on health and the huge volumes of genomic data available on the web relating to the noncoding genome. Although we cannot claim that all of the data available is easy to access, we would encourage anybody who seeks to understand the role of epigenetics in health and disease to engage with these databases in order to inform their future experimental decisions. Many research institutes and universities also now employ dedicated bioinformaticians who would be willing to help and expand on the content of this chapter. In addition, NCBI, USCS, and ENSEMBL also have dedicated and largely underused help desks which are able to rapidly inform and facilitate use of their respective databases.

We will initially introduce the noncoding genome and the "zoo" of different elements within it, which are known to regulate the expression of genes essential to health. We will then briefly examine the different types of epigenetic modification and describe how these different modifications affect the activity of noncoding gene regulatory elements. We will then describe how we can use online data mining of existing databases to identify functional regions of the genome affected by epigenetic modification and how these modifications might interact with polymorphic variation. The noncoding genome encompasses all regulatory DNA (cis- and trans-regions) as well as nonfunctional DNA sequences. This chapter will focus on the cis-regulatory genome and it is intended to provide an insight into how to access these databases to facilitate an understanding of how variation in the genome may interact with environmentally induced epigenetic modifications to maintain health through life, and alter disease susceptibility and possibly drug responses.

1.1 Types of Epigenetic Modification

1.1.1 DNA Methylation

Methylation of CpG islands has been shown to play a significant role in disease states such as cardiovascular disease, obesity, and type 2 diabetes [2–4]. Environmental factors such as stress can alter DNA methylation and have been linked to the onset of mental illnesses [5]. Tobacco exposure has also been shown to cause hypomethylation of oncogene promoters and hypermethylation of tumor suppressor gene promoters, providing a possible mechanism for the development of cancer [6]. DNA methylation occurs when a methyl group is transferred to carbon 5 of the purine or pyrimidine ring of a DNA base by an enzyme from the family of DNA methyltransferases [6]. Most DNA methylation occurs at cysteine residues present in CpG dinucleotides. DNA methylation is known to alter gene expression. For example, gene silencing via the methylation of CpG islands contained within promoters can lead to altered cell signaling pathways [7]. Approximately half of all CpG islands are associated with promoter regions [8] and 72 % of the promoters of annotated genes have been found to have a high CpG content compared to the rest of the genome [9]. However, many CpG-rich promoters are maintained in a hypomethylated state which may be due to secondary folding of the DNA containing CpG islands [10]. There are several proposed mechanisms of altering transcription by DNA methylation. Transcription factors may be prevented from binding to their target sequences in promoters due to DNA methylation at these sites or be blocked by proteins such as MECP2 MBD1, MBD2, MBD3, and MBD4, which bind to methylated DNA [11]. See note 1 for information on analyzing this type of data on genome browsers.

1.1.2 Chromatin Modification

Histone acetylation and methylation are two different types of chromatin modifications that, together, modulate what has become known as the Histone Code. Indeed, there are so many identified histone modifications that it is theoretically possible for each nucleosome within the genome to have its own unique histone signature. For example, histone acetylation is controlled by two types of enzymes, histone acetyltransferases (HATs) which transfer acetyl groups to the ε-amino group of the lysine residue, and histone deacetylases (HDACs) which remove acetyl groups [12]. Acetyl groups neutralize the positive charge of lysine [12]. As DNA is negatively charged, this results in a weaker interaction between chromatin, giving a more open chromatin conformation (euchromatin). Varying the level of acetylation therefore alters the availability of DNA for transcription factor binding. In most cases, lysine acetylation corresponds to the activation of gene transcription [6]. Methylation of lysine is another common form of histone modification, which can be in the form of mono-methyl, di-methyl, and tri-methyl groups added to histone proteins by the group of methyltransferase enzymes. Different epigenetic markers have been identified with different states of gene transcription. For example, mono-, di-, and tri-methylation of lysine 4 on histone 3 (H3K4) are indicative of active promoters whilst H3K9 di- and tri-methylation are indicative of repressed promoters [12].

1.2 Epigenetics and Gene Regulation

1.2.1 Promoters

It is becoming clearer that one of the most important ways that epigenetic modification affects the genome and impacts health is by altering the activity of gene regulatory regions. The best characterized gene regulatory regions are promoters. The promoter is a region of DNA next to the transcriptional start site of genes that acts as the point of assembly of the core transcriptional apparatus, also known as the preinitiation complex (PIC), which includes RNA polymerase II. A key characteristic of promoters is that they are distance and orientation dependant with respect to the transcriptional start site (TSS) of the genes they control. The preinitiation complex (PIC; includes TFII proteins, RNApolII, and mediator) is assembled on the core promoter, which is approximately 80 bases in length [13]. However promoters have been erroneously described as being many more kilobases longer than this, and therefore these "promoters" are likely to contain the core promoter as well as other proximal cis-regulatory elements which influence the promoter, such as enhancers and silencers.

1.2.2 The Encyclopedia of DNA Elements (ENCODE) Consortium

ENCODE is a project which aims to reveal and characterize the functional elements of the human genome. The ENCODE consortium suggested that approximately 80 % of the genome has a function [14]. This observation is contentious however, as only 10 % of the genome has been shown to be under selective pressure [15]. Nevertheless, ENCODE also demonstrated that there may be around 4.5 times more regulatory DNA than coding DNA [14]. The relevance of this noncoding information is supported by the observation that the majority (71 %) of GWAS disease-associated single nucleotide polymorphisms (SNPs) occur in regulatory elements [14], thus highlighting the importance of studying these regions for a greater understanding of disease, differences in drug efficacy, and for developing personalized medicines. Furthermore, these regions are also susceptible to epigenetic modifications, which include DNA methylation and histone modifications.

The University of California Santa Cruz (UCSC) genome browser [16] provides access to data produced by the ENCODE consortium and can be used to identify promoter regions using specific histone marks and a number of other techniques such as DNAseI-seq and formaldehyde assisted isolation of regulatory elements (FAIRE) analysis. Data from other projects are also available on this browser. It is therefore a useful starting point for finding putative cis-regulatory regions and their associated SNPs and epigenetic modifications. The National Centre for Biotechnology Information (NCBI) provides access to functional genomic studies from which data can be downloaded and superimposed onto data in UCSC genome browser for analysis. NCBI also provides a tool for further analysis of SNPs found on the UCSC genome browser such as their allelic population proportions.

1.2.3 Cis-regulatory Elements

Cis-regulatory elements are noncoding regions of the genome which are responsible for regulating gene transcription by communicating cellular signals to gene promoters [17]. Cis-regulatory regions include enhancers, silencers, and insulator sequences. There are several detection protocols that have been developed for identifying cis-regulatory regions. Chromatin immunoprecipitation (ChIP) assays have been developed to identify DNA sequences associated with specific histone modifications or the binding of proteins. In addition, FAIRE-seq and DNAse1 sensitivity mapping (DNAse-seq) assays detect open chromatin configurations in the genome [18].

ChIP-seq analyses histone modifications and the binding of transcription factors and histone proteins to genomic DNA. Cells are cultured and treated with formaldehyde to cross-link the protein to the DNA by covalent bonding. Sonication is often used to fragment the chromatin. The protein of interest is detected by applying a specific antibody, conjugated to beads which can be separated by centrifugation or using magnets. Following washing to remove non-bound chromatin and reversal of cross-links, next-generation sequencing of the immunoprecipitated DNA allows for determining the level of interaction of transcription factor or modified histone throughout the genome of the cell line under analysis.

DNAse-seq and FAIRE-seq both involve degradation of transcriptionally active DNA. That is DNA which is not associated with nucleosomes where chromatin is said to be in an open configuration. DNAse-seq uses the enzyme DNAse1 which penetrates the nuclei of lysed cells and degrades DNA in the open configuration. The digested DNA is then recovered and undergoes next-generation sequencing. FAIRE-seq uses formaldehyde to cross-link proteins to DNA. Therefore, following sonication and phenol extraction, exposed DNA which is not cross-linked to nucleosomes will be separated into the aqueous phase whilst DNA firmly linked to nucleosomes will separate into the phenol phase. The DNA recovered from the aqueous phase therefore undergoes next-generation sequencing.

These techniques have been effective and reliable in identifying transcriptionally open and active chromatin and in the cell lines used by ENCODE. Whilst these techniques identify transcriptionally active regions, such as promoters and enhancers, other techniques developed from chromatin conformation capture (3C) assays can identify interactions between regions of DNA which are several hundred kilobases apart, but which are proximate to each other when chromatin loops to bring enhancers and promoters together. 3C can identify looping in DNA which results in long-distance DNA interactions [19]. The technique uses formaldehyde initially, to cross-link interacting DNA loci with bound proteins regulating the interaction. Subsequent restriction endonuclease digestion breaks the chromatin into small fragments which are then subjected to circularization with DNA ligase and tagged nucleotides. The interacting sequences are identified by PCR, using locus-specific primers [20]. From this technique, carbon copy 3C (5C) and HiC have been developed that use next-generation sequencing techniques to allow for genome-wide identification of interacting DNA regions.

1.2.4 Comparative Genomics

Comparative genomics utilizes the hypothesis that genomic sequences that play a critical role in species fitness and survival are conserved through evolutionary time whereas regions of the genome that are relatively unimportant change over time due to natural genetic drift. Whilst this approach has clearly identified the importance of sequence integrity in gene coding regions for survival, comparative genomics has also succeeded in identifying a huge portion of the genome that does not encode protein but which has been hugely conserved nevertheless. Recovery of highly conserved noncoding sequences has been used successfully on a number of occasions to identify novel tissue-specific cis-regulatory sequences. However, the application of comparative genomics to identify cis-regulatory regions has been largely overshadowed by the use of whole genome next-generation sequence (NGS)-based ChIP-seq, FAIRE, and DNase-seq methodologies as typified by ENCODE. Whilst the use of these NGS-based methods represent a "snapshot" of the protein-DNA interactions within a specific cell line, they are unable to identify regulatory regions of the genome that are critical to survival in all cells of an organisms, under all conditions and at all stages of their life cycle. Only comparative genomics can come near to achieving this goal as many cis-regulatory regions critical for survival may only be active within specific cells and under very specific circumstances. Thus, an enhancer such as GAL5.1 that has been implicated in controlling the expression of the galanin neuropeptide in a tiny group of cells within the peri-ventricular nucleus of the hypothalamus, where galanin controls fat and alcohol intake, is almost invisible to ENCODE and can only be identified by virtue of its extreme evolutionary conservation [21]. Indeed, a recent study of p300 protein binding, a characteristic of active enhancer regions, in primary cells of E10.5 mouse embryos has shown that there is a much tighter correlation between enhancers and conserved regions of the genome [22]. Probably the greatest advantage from a practical point of view is that comparative genomics is easy and very accessible thanks to the availability of whole genome sequence from over 100 vertebrates available through the UCSC browser.

1.3 Accessing the Genome Browser

The UCSC genome browser provides access to the genomes of a wide range of different species as well as several assemblies of the human genome. The most recent assembly is GRCh38/hg38 which was completed in December 2013. However for the examples provided in this chapter GRCh37/hg19 is used which was completed in February 2009. This is because the genomic annotations associated with each assembly take time to be fully transferred and updated. Thus, GRCh37/hg19 will be described here as it provides a more extensive annotation of the human genome including regulatory regions.

2 Materials

The UCSC Genome Bioinformatics web site: http://genome-euro. ucsc.edu/index.html

National Centre for Biotechnology Information web site: http://www.ncbi.nlm.nih.gov

Methods for downloading GEO Data: http://www.ncbi.nlm.nih.gov/geo/info/download.html

Ensemble database: http://www.ensembl.org/index.html

Array Express: http://www.ebi.ac.uk/arrayexpress/

3 Methods

3.1 Identifying Cis-regulatory Regions

1. Go to web site address http://genome-euro.ucsc.edu/index.html (This is the European mirror for the UCSC genome. Users based in the States will have automatic access to the US site) and select **Genome Browser** at the top of the left-hand panel.

2. Select the **Group**, **Genome**, and **Assembly** that you would like to study and enter the position (in coordinates) or the gene name that you wish to search for in the **search term box** and click **Submit**.

3. You will be asked to select a transcript variant.

4. A screen similar to the following will be shown (Fig. 1). See note 2 for details of features shown in Fig. 1.

5. Scrolling down will show tracks that allow for further analysis of the gene. The first subdivision (Mapping and sequencing), shown in Fig. 2, shows mapping and basic sequence data such as GC percentages, Sequence tagged site (STS) markers, and restriction endonuclease cut sites. Symbols resembling two stacked X shapes represent data derived from the ENCODE consortium dataset.

6. One of the default tracks is the conservation track, shown in green in Fig. 1. Using comparative genomics, this track shows conservation of sequences throughout over 100 vertebrates. This track can be altered by clicking **Conservation** under the comparative genomics heading shown in Fig. 3, to include a large volume of organisms spanning primates to jawless fishes that represents an evolutionary distance of some 450 million years. These tracks are especially useful for identifying

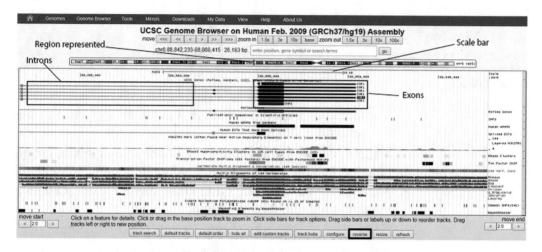

Fig. 1 A typical display shown following a search for a specific gene in the UCSC genome browser. This image will vary depending on the gene searched for, the set magnification of the image (altered by zoom), and the default track settings. Image taken from http:/genome.ucsc.edu [16]

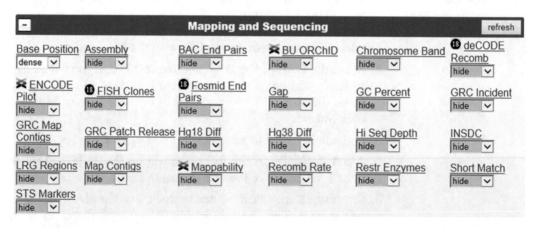

Fig. 2 The Mapping and Sequencing tracks available in the UCSC genome browser. BU ORChid, ENCODE pilot, and Mappability are tracks which show data from the ENCODE consortium. Image taken from http:/genome.ucsc.edu [16]

Fig. 3 Comparative genomics tracks in the UCSC genome browser, which include the Conservation track. Image taken from http:/genome.ucsc.edu [16]

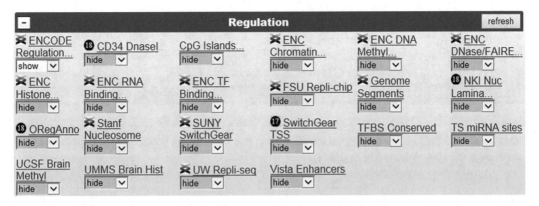

Fig. 4 Regulation tracks, in the UCSC genome browser, which are useful for analyzing the regulatory genome and epigenetic modifications. Image taken from http:/genome.ucsc.edu [16]

important regions of both the coding and noncoding genome by virtue of their evolutionary conservation.

7. Tracks under the **Regulation** heading, shown in Fig. 4, are especially useful for analyzing the regulatory genome and epigenetic targets. Sections 3.2–3.6 will focus on the **Regulation** tracks.

8. More information about the tracks as well as subtracks (if applicable) and display settings can be found by clicking on each of the track headings (See note 3 for more information about the regulatory genome).

3.2 Promoters

The use of comparative genomics has greatly advanced the detection of conserved noncoding, cis-regulatory regions, which are therefore likely to have a function. More specifically, different markers of promoters can be detected and used to indicate the activity of the promoter.

1. CpG islands, diagnostic of many promoter regions, can be identified using the **CpG Islands** track. Methylated cytosines are more susceptible to spontaneous deamination to become thymines; therefore, the presence of CpG islands indicate that they have been conserved and have a function. The proto-oncogene, *MYC*, is represented in Fig. 5, where CpG islands are shown in green.

2. The **ENCODE Histone Modification** track reflects ChIP-seq-based analyses to determine modifications to particular residues of histones within the nucleosomes making up the chromatin at any specific position. Specific histone modifications such as H3K4me3 are indicative of the activity of the promoter (*see* Fig. 6). See note 4 about using different display conventions. See note 5 for more information about analyzing epigenetic modifications.

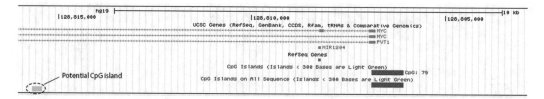

Fig. 5 CpG islands associated with the *Myc* gene are shown in green. The "CpG Islands on All Sequence" track includes potential CpG islands associated with the gene; this function can be selected in the track settings. Image taken from http:/genome.ucsc.edu [16]

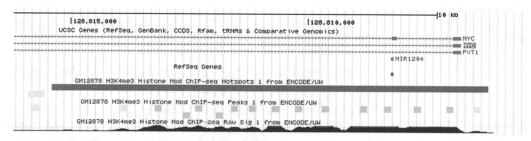

Fig. 6 The H3K4Me3 modification at the *MYC* gene within GM12878 cells. This histone modification is indicative of active promoters. Image taken from http:/genome.ucsc.edu [16]

3.3 Transcription Factor Binding

1. The **ENCODE transcription factor binding** tracks indicate transcription factor binding sites which have been discovered using the ChIP-seq technique. Transcription factors are indicated on the right-hand side of the tracks next to the names of the cell lines in which the ChIP-seq analysis was carried out (e.g., GM12878 CTCF). For example CTCF binding sites, which are accepted diagnostics of insulator sequences, can be displayed by selecting the desired display mode from the UW CTCF binding track and open chromatin transcription factor binding sites can be displayed using the UTA TFBS track. An example of the cell lines which can be selected and the UTA TFBS track is shown in Fig. 7.

2. The **TFBS (Transcription Factor Binding Site) conserved** track uses transcription factor binding motifs predicted by the TRANSFAC database [23] to predict conserved transcription factor binding sites across the mouse, rat, and human genomes (Fig. 8).

3.4 Transcriptional Regulation

1. The **ENCODE regulation** track shows information related to regulation of transcription based on the collated data derived from the cell lines used. The transcription subtrack shows transcription levels in different cell types (*see* **Note 6**). Clicking on the subtrack will provide a list of the cell types studied and their color codes. Other subtracks provide information

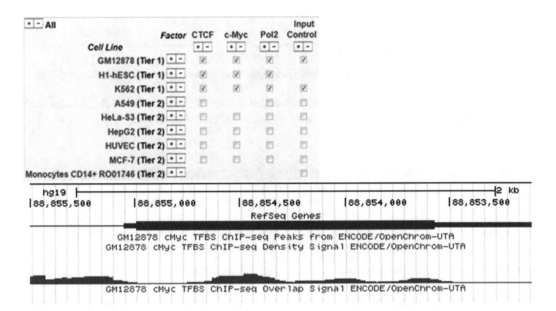

Fig. 7 Some of the cell lines and transcription factors which can be selected (*top*) and an example of open chromatin transcription factor binding sites on the *CNR1* gene (*bottom*). Image taken from http:/genome.ucsc.edu [16]

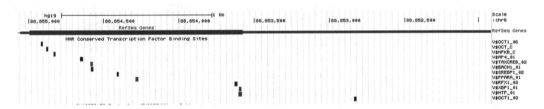

Fig. 8 Conserved transcription factor binding sites for *CNR1* are shown by *black boxes*. Transcription factor binding sites are labeled on the *right-hand side* of the screen. Clicking on a *black box* gives more information, such as a list of transcription factors that bind to the site. Image taken from http:/genome.ucsc.edu [16]

regarding histone modifications indicative of enhancer or promoter regions and regions of chromatin which are sensitive to DNase. An example of transcription levels is shown in Fig. 9.

2. The **ENCODE Open Chromatin by DNaseI HS and FAIRE Tracks** provide information from ENCODE about open chromatin which is indicative of DNA which is accessible by transcription factors or other regulatory molecules due to removal of nucleosomes (combination of genomic DNA and histones). To investigate chromatin configuration DNAse hypersensitivity, FAIRE and ChIP assays were used. This has been assessed in various cell types and tissues.

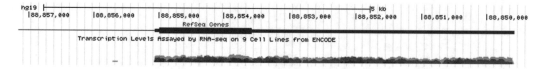

Fig. 9 Transcription levels for the *CNR1* gene. The display convention selected was **Full**. Different colors represent different cell types assayed. Image taken from http:/genome.ucsc.edu [16]

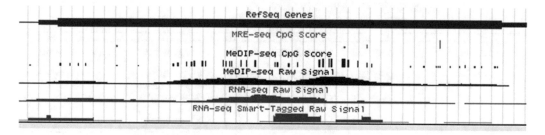

Fig. 10 Brain DNA methylation of *CNR1*. The different techniques employed are indicated on each track. Immunoprecipitation is employed to identify methylated regions in MeDIP-seq. Unmethylated CpGs are identified by MRE-seq. Image taken from http:/genome.ucsc.edu [16]

3. The **Genome segments** track suggests a function for specific regions of the genome based on an analysis of the encode data derived from tier 1 and tier 2 cell lines. Each type of region is color coded. The color key can be found by clicking on the track headings. For example, green represents predicted transcribed regions, grey represents predicted repressed or low activity regions, and yellow represents predicted weak enhancer regions or cis-regulatory regions in open chromatin.

3.5 DNA Methylation

1. The **ENCODE DNA methylation** tracks provide information about DNA methylation on the gene of interest. The cell types that this was tested in are shown on the right-hand side (e.g., HUVEC, GM12878). One method of detecting DNA methylation is by bisulphite sequencing which converts unmethylated cysteines to uracil leaving methylated cysteines to be detected. Other methods used to assess methylation include MeDIP (Methylated DNA immunoprecipitation) and MRE (Methylation sensitive Restriction endonuclease digestion) that are shown in the UCSF Brain Methylation track.

2. The **UCSF Brain DNA methylation** track shows human DNA methylation patterns in postmortem frontal cortex of a 57-year-old male. Several methods were employed. For example, the H3K4me3 modification was detected by ChIP-seq. An example of brain DNA methylation at *CNR1* is shown in Fig. 10.

3.6 Long-Distance Chromatin Interactions

1. Long range genomic interactions detected by derivatives of chromatin conformation capture (3C) analysis that use next-generation sequencing such as 5C can be viewed using the **ENCODE Chromatin Interaction** tracks.

2. Two different subtracks can be selected, one for chromatin interactions discovered by 5C and one which used the chromatin interaction analysis by paired-end tag (ChIA-PET) technique.

3.7 Single Nucleotide Polymorphisms

1. Under the **Variation** heading, the **Common SNPs** track is useful for finding more information on SNPs found in 1 % or more of the human population. An example of this track is shown in Fig. 11. More information about the display conventions of the SNPs can be found by clicking the track heading.

2. By clicking on an SNP of interest, information about the SNP can be found such as the reference allele and the alleles found in other species.

3. Clicking dbSNP takes you to the National Centre for Biotechnology (NCBI) Information web site which provides information about allelic proportions within populations.

3.8 Additional Tools, Genome Browsers, and Databases

In addition to analyzing data provided by the UCSC genome browser, you can upload your own data to the browser to analyze. This data will only be available temporarily, on the computer that it was uploaded from.

1. Firstly, your data files must be published as web pages to the central staff pages system of your institute's web server.

2. On the genome browser home page, the corresponding organism should be selected, followed by clicking on **add custom tracks**, indicated in Fig. 12.

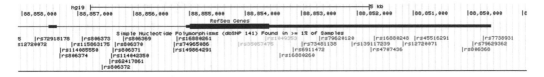

Fig. 11 Common SNPs identified in the *CNR1* gene. Image taken from http:/genome.ucsc.edu [16]

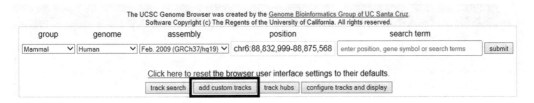

Fig. 12 The UCSC genome browser search page. The **add custom tracks** button is *highlighted*. Image taken from http:/genome.ucsc.edu [16]

3. The URL of your published data files can then be pasted into the box provided.

4. More details on this tool, including the file formats supported by the browser, can be found at http://genome.ucsc.edu/goldenpath/help/customTrack.html.

Similarly, files from other databases can be uploaded to the UCSC genome browser for analysis. For example, the Gene Expression Omnibus (GEO) database [24] on the NCBI web site provides access to data from high-throughput functional genomic studies for free.

1. By going to http://www.ncbi.nlm.nih.gov and selecting GEO databases (Fig. 13), you can search using keywords such as a disease, organism, or gene.

2. Geo datasets can be downloaded by several methods, including creating a URL, and these methods are explained at http://www.ncbi.nlm.nih.gov/geo/info/download.html.

3. Other databases are also available for viewing and analyzing data. For example Ensembl (found at http://www.ensembl.org/index.html) [25] also provides data produced by the ENCODE project and also allows upload of your own data.

4. ArrayExpress (found at http://www.ebi.ac.uk/arrayexpress/) [26] is provided by the European Bioinformatics Institute and, similarly to NCBI, provides data from functional genomics studies. Following a keyword search, results can be filtered by organism, array, and/or experiment type. An example search is shown in Fig. 14.

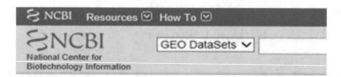

Fig. 13 Geo datasets should be selected from this drop-down menu to search for data from high-throughput functional genomic studies. Image taken from http://www.ncbi.nlm.nih.gov/

ArrayExpress results for *"diabetes mellitus"*   + Show more data from EMBL-EBI

Accession	Title	Type	Organism	Assays	Released	Processed	Raw	Atlas
E-MTAB-3070	Gene expression profiling of MafA, MafB, and MafA/MafB Mutants in E18.5 pancreas	transcription profiling by array	Mus musculus	15	04/11/2014	±	±	-
E-GEOD-62390	Staphylococcus aureus gene expression in a rat model of infective endocarditis	transcription profiling by array	Staphylococcus aureus	9	01/11/2014	±	±	-
E-GEOD-57896	White-to-brown metabolic conversion of human adipocytes by JAK inhibition	RNA-seq of coding RNA	Homo sapiens	30	31/10/2014	-	-	-
E-GEOD-54374	An integrated cell purification and genomics strategy reveals multiple regulators of pancreas development.	transcription profiling by array	Mus musculus	48	16/10/2014	±	±	-

Fig. 14 An example search on ArrayExpress. The search can be filtered using the drop-down menus in the lilac box. Image taken from http://www.ebi.ac.uk/arrayexpress/ [26]

4 Notes

1. When analyzing data from genome browsers, the techniques used to generate the data must be considered. For example, bisulfite conversion sequencing cannot differentiate between the production of 5-methyl-cytosine (5mC) by enzymes DNMT3A and DNMT3B, a marker of transcriptionally repressed chromatin, and the production of 5-hydroxymethyl-cytosine (5hmC) by the TET enzyme, a marker of active enhancers and promoters [27, 28]. However, a newly developed technique of oxidative bisulfite sequencing is capable of distinguishing between these two forms of methylation [29].

2. The scale bar at the top of the view in Fig. 1 demonstrates the size of the region of the genome being displayed. Grey buttons at the top allows the user to zoom in or out or move along the sequence in either direction. A search box allows the user to input gene names, single nucleotide polymorphism (SNP numbers (rs-No.)), or genomic coordinates (e.g., chr6:88,575, 853-88,854,993) to search the human genome. Default tracks are shown underneath however; these can be removed by right-clicking on them and selecting **hide**. Other options are also given, when right-clicking, to allow you to change how the track is viewed and the configuration. For example, clicking **Full** will show each feature of the track on an independent line whereas **Pack** will label each feature. The chromosome is shown with a red line indicating the position of the region represented in the box. Chevrons on the transcript indicate the direction of transcription. By clicking the **reverse** button underneath the browser will orientate the gene in the opposite direction. The lines decorated with arrow heads indicate intronic regions (arrows indicate the direction of transcription), and filled black boxes show the exons, with thicker boxes indicative of coding regions and thinner boxes indicative of untranslated regions. All known splice forms of the gene mRNA are also indicated. Splice variants can also be viewed with ACEview or GENCODE annotation tracks which also show conserved coding regions (CDSs) and polyadenylation (poly-A) sites.

3. Genome-wide genetic association studies have shown that non-coding regions of DNA contain up to 93 % of SNPs associated with disease, with 73 % of these being present in regions thought to have regulatory function [30]. This highlights the importance in researching these regions with regard to disease, contradicting the perception that noncoding regions are "junk" DNA.

4. Different display conventions can be selected from the track settings. An example is shown in Fig. 6 for the *MYC* gene.

Only the **UW Histone** track was selected in this example and the display was set as **Pack**.

5. We must accept the possibility that the significance of association data derived from candidate locus analysis or even GWA analysis in humans is affected by differences in epigenetic profiles within patient cohorts. Thus, the penetrance of the phenotypic effects of an allelic variant may be masked or exacerbated by epigenetic factors such as CpG methylation or histone modification. Indeed, the interaction of epigenetics with genetic variation in the preservation of health and the exacerbation of disease may be a confounding factor in the majority of candidate and genome-wide association analyses that requires further analysis.

6. Although prediction of cis-regulatory elements using the techniques employed by major genome-wide data repositories such as ENCODE is largely based on observations derived from cancer cell lines and embryonic stem cells that may differ considerably from cells in vivo, ENCODE are continuously updating their databases with data derived from much more representative cell types. Therefore, it is essential that these databases are revisited as often as possible to take advantage of the latest data releases.

Acknowledgements

We would like to thank Dr. Susan Fairley from the University of Aberdeen for providing information about other genome browsers and databases mentioned in Section 3.8. Elizabeth A. Hay is funded by Medical Research Scotland (PhD-719-2013) and GW Pharmaceuticals. Philip Cowie was funded by the Scottish Universities Life Science Alliance (SULCA).

References

1. Tost J (2010) DNA methylation: an introduction to the biology and the disease-associated changes of a promising biomarker. Mol Biotechnol 44(1):71–81

2. Tarry-Adkins JL, Ozanne SE (2014) The impact of early nutrition on the ageing trajectory. Proc Nutr Soc 73:289

3. Glier MB, Green TJ, Devlin AM (2013) Methyl nutrients, DNA methylation, and cardiovascular disease. Mol Nutr Food Res 58(1):172–182

4. Drummond EM, Gibney ER (2013) Epigenetic regulation in obesity. Curr Opin Clin Nutr Metab Care 16(4):392–397

5. Dalton VS, Kolshus E, McLoughlin DM (2013) Epigenetics and depression: return of the repressed. J Affect Disord 155:1–12

6. Armstrong L (2014) Epigenetics, 1st edn. Garland science, New York

7. Jin B, Robertson KD (2012) DNA methyltransferases, DNA damage repair, and cancer. Adv Exp Med Biol 754:3–29

8. Deaton AM et al (2011) CpG islands and the regulation of transcription. Genes Dev 25(10):1010–1022

9. Saxonov S et al (2006) A genome-wide analysis of CpG dinucleotides in the human genome

distinguishes two distinct classes of promoters. Proc Natl Acad Sci U S A 103(5):1412–1417

10. Ginno PA et al (2012) R-loop formation is a distinctive characteristic of unmethylated human CpG island promoters. Mol Cell 45 (6):814–825

11. Moore LD, Le T, Fan G (2012) DNA methylation and its basic function. Neuropsychopharmacology 38(1):23–38

12. Bannister AJ, Kouzarides T (2011) Regulation of chromatin by histone modifications. Cell Res 21(3):381–395

13. Juven-Gershon T, Kadonaga JT (2009) Regulation of gene expression via the core promoter and the basal transcriptional machinery. Dev Biol 339(2):225–229

14. Dunham I et al (2012) An integrated encyclopedia of DNA elements in the human genome. Nature 489(7414):57–74

15. Graur D et al (2013) On the immortality of television sets: "function" in the human genome according to the evolution-free gospel of ENCODE. Genome Biol Evol 5 (3):578–590

16. Kent WJ et al (2002) The human genome browser at UCSC. Genome Res 12(6):996–1006

17. MacKenzie A, Hing B, Davidson S (2013) Exploring the effects of polymorphisms on cis-regulatory signal transduction response. Trends Mol Med 19(2):99–107

18. Song L et al (2011) Open chromatin defined by DNaseI and FAIRE identifies regulatory elements that shape cell-type identity. Genome Res 21(10):1757–1767

19. Dekker J et al (2002) Capturing chromosome conformation. Science 295(5558):1306–1311

20. Gheldof N, Leleu M, Noordermeer D, Rougemont J, Reymond A (2012) Detecting long-range chromatin interactions using the chromosome conformation capture sequencing (4C-seq) method*. In: Deplancke B, Gheldof N (eds) Gene regulatory networks, Methods and protocols. Humana Press, Totowa, NJ

21. Davidson S et al (2011) Differential activity by polymorphic variants of a remote enhancer that supports galanin expression in the hypothalamus and amygdala: implications for obesity. Depression and alcoholism. Neuropsychopharmacology 36:2211–2221

22. Visel A et al (2009) ChIP-seq accurately predicts tissue-specific activity of enhancers. Nature 457(7231):854–858

23. Matys V et al (2006) TRANSFAC and its module TRANSCompel: transcriptional gene regulation in eukaryotes. Nucleic Acids Res 34 (Database issue):D108–D110

24. Edgar R, Domrachev M, Lash AE (2002) Gene expression omnibus: NCBI gene expression and hybridization array data repository. Nucleic Acids Res 30(1):207–210

25. Cunningham F et al (2015) Ensembl 2015. Nucleic Acids Res 43(D1):D662–D669

26. Kolesnikov N et al (2015) ArrayExpress update - simplifying data submissions. Nucleic Acids Res 43(Database issue):D1113–D1116

27. Branco MR, Ficz G, Reik W (2011) Uncovering the role of 5-hydroxymethylcytosine in the epigenome. Nat Rev Genet 13(1):7–13

28. Ficz G et al (2011) Dynamic regulation of 5-hydroxymethylcytosine in mouse ES cells and during differentiation. Nature 473 (7347):398–402

29. Booth MJ et al (2013) Oxidative bisulfite sequencing of 5-methylcytosine and 5-hydroxymethylcytosine. Nat Protoc 8 (10):1841–1851

30. Maurano MT et al (2012) Systematic localization of common disease-associated variation in regulatory DNA. Science 337(6099): 1190–1195

Methods in Molecular Biology (2017) 1589: 47–74
DOI 10.1007/7651_2015_261
© Springer Science+Business Media New York 2016
Published online: 23 February 2016

Detecting Spatial Chromatin Organization by Chromosome Conformation Capture II: Genome-Wide Profiling by Hi-C

Matteo Vietri Rudan, Suzana Hadjur, and Tom Sexton

Abstract

The chromosome conformation capture (3C) method has been invaluable in studying chromatin interactions in a population of cells at a resolution surpassing that of light microscopy, for example in the detection of functional contacts between enhancers and promoters. Recent developments in sequencing-based chromosomal contact mapping (Hi-C, 5C and 4C-Seq) have allowed researchers to interrogate pairwise chromatin interactions on a wider scale, shedding light on the three-dimensional organization of chromosomes. These methods present significant technical and bioinformatic challenges to consider at the start of the project. Here, we describe two alternative methods for Hi-C, depending on the size of the genome, and discuss the major computational approaches to convert the raw sequencing data into meaningful models of how genomes are organized.

Keywords: Hi-C, 3C (chromosome conformation capture), Chromatin interactions, Chromosome topology, High-throughput sequencing

1 Introduction

Chromosomes must be densely packaged in order to fit into nuclear space. Microscopy techniques have firmly established that chromosomes are nonrandomly organized within the nucleus and that this organization is intimately linked to genome function [1]. Despite these important advances, microscopy methods are limited in their resolution and throughput and thus a comprehensive understanding of chromosome structure has been lacking.

Chromosome conformation capture (3C) is a molecular biology approach that allows the physical proximity of two genomic sites to be assessed in vivo at significantly higher resolution than can be obtained by microscopy, and was first used to describe the three-dimensional conformation of a yeast chromosome [2]. Briefly, the method involves fixation of chromatin in its native state (primarily using formaldehyde), followed by restriction digestion of the fixed chromatin and subsequent re-ligation of the cut chromatin under conditions favoring intramolecular ligation. This generates hybrid DNA restriction fragments comprised of sequences which may have been very far away from one another in linear distance, but which were physically proximal at the time of fixation and therefore "captured" as ligation events [2, 3].

Since the advent of the 3C method, various genomic derivatives of the technique have been developed and have greatly refined previous models of chromosome organization [4]. Among these, the Hi-C method allows for the simultaneous detection of all possible interactions [5]. Recent Hi-C studies have shown that metazoan genomes contain discretely folded modules of high contact intensity, referred to as "topological domains" [6, 7]. These domains encompass multiple genes and overlap extensively with active and repressive epigenetic marks. This important discovery characterizes a missing link in chromosomal biology, embedding thousands of genes and enhancers into large mammalian chromosomes in a meaningful and structured way. Hi-C has also been used to probe the functional roles of domains and the factors which define domain borders and their internal structures [8–10].

The strength of Hi-C in globally assessing *all* possible chromatin interactions also creates its own challenges, namely the number of possible products that can be captured is much greater than current sequencing outputs will detect. For example, the human genome consists of ~1.7 million HindIII fragments, resulting in ~1.4×10^{12} possible pairwise combinations of 3C ligation products. As a consequence, most Hi-C interaction matrices are probabilistic rather than quantitative (i.e., a specific long-range interaction between two restriction fragments is scored as present or absent, rather than counted). Summing multiple discretely detected interactions is necessary to obtain statistical confidence, whether by looking at all features simultaneously (e.g., contact insulation around all cohesin/CTCF co-bound sites) [9] or by studying interactions at lower resolution with windows encompassing multiple restriction fragments [8]. While Hi-C is the principal method for global studies of chromatin architecture, researchers may want to consider more focused 3C variants, such as 4C-seq [11], if they require high-resolution, semi-quantitative interaction profiles of a limited subset of genomic loci.

Here we describe two alternative ways of performing Hi-C. The first simply involves paired-end sequencing of 3C material and was used to obtain the chromatin interactome of *Drosophila melanogaster* embryos [7]. This method is easy to do and requires minimal optimization; it is described here for Drosophila embryos. However, a lot of sequences are obtained which are uninformative about chromatin interactions, such as self-ligation events, and need to be discarded; prohibitively large numbers of sequence reads are required to usefully apply this technique to larger, metazoan genomes such as human. The second Hi-C method described here, originally applied to human cells [5], removes these uninformative reads by including a preselection for true 3C ligation events. Briefly, chromatin is digested as in a conventional 3C experiment, but the cohesive ends of digested fragments are filled in with biotinylated nucleotides by DNA polymerase before ligation of blunt ends. The incorporated biotinylated nucleotide allows the library to be enriched for ligation junctions before library sequencing. The method is described here for primary mouse hepatocytes. It should be noted that the basic 3C methods described are different due to their optimization for different tissues; extended information on optimizing the 3C protocol can be found in another chapter [3]. The output of both methods is a catalog of paired-end sequences which includes both putative chromatin interactions and nonfunctional interactions. We will also discuss the computational steps to filter the initial sequencing files, generate models of background interactions, and obtain normalized chromatin interaction maps.

2 Materials

2.1 Hi-C Method 1: Direct Sequencing of 3C Material in Drosophila Embryos

1. Embryo collection cages and sieve collection system.

2. Plates of Drosophila egg-laying medium plates (agar plus 15 % vinegar, 1 % methylparaben and Neutral Red dye), coated with yeast. Melt 8.75 g agar in 275 ml water in a microwave, add 48 ml vinegar, 3.2 ml methylparaben, and a pinch of Neutral Red, then autoclave. Medium can be stored at 4 °C for a few weeks. Melt the medium in a microwave, pour into petri dishes, and leave to set. Plates can be stored at 4 °C for a few days. Just before use, coat a paste of yeast onto the plate.

3. Embryo collection buffer: 0.4 % (w/v) NaCl, 0.03 % (v/v) Triton-X100.

4. Bleach.

5. Drosophila fixation buffer: 2 % formaldehyde (*see* **Note 1**), 15 mM HEPES pH 7.6, 60 mM KCl, 15 mM NaCl, 4 mM MgCl$_2$, 0.1 % Triton-X100, 0.5 mM DTT, EDTA-free protease inhibitor cocktail (Roche). Buffer is made fresh on the day of use from the stocks of the individual components; formaldehyde and protease inhibitor cocktail are added just prior to fixation.

6. 7 ml Toenbroeck douncer.

7. Temperature-controlled shaker, with adapters for 1.5 ml microcentrifuge tubes, 15 ml falcon tubes, and 50 ml falcon tubes.

8. 2 M glycine.

9. Drosophila wash buffer: Fixation buffer without formaldehyde. Buffer is made fresh on the day of use from the stocks of individual components and stored on ice prior to use.

10. 1.25× NEB3 buffer: 125 mM NaCl, 62.5 mM Tris–HCl pH 8, 12.5 mM MgCl$_2$, 1.25 mM DTT. Buffer is made fresh on the

day of use from stocks of individual components and stored on ice prior to use.

11. 1.25× DpnII buffer. Buffer is made from 10× stock provided by NEB (*see* **Note 2**).

12. 20 % SDS.

13. 20 % Triton-X100.

14. High-concentration DpnII (50,000 U/ml; NEB) (*see* **Notes 2** and **3**).

15. Drosophila ligation buffer: 1× T4 DNA ligase buffer (made from 10× stock from NEB), 1 % Triton-X100. Buffer is made fresh on the day of use.

16. High-concentration T4 DNA ligase (2,000,000 U/ml; NEB).

17. 10 mg/ml proteinase K.

18. 20 mg/ml RNase A.

19. Undersaturated phenol solution: 90 % undersaturated phenol, 100 mM Tris base, 10 mM 8-hydroxyquinoline. Melt undersaturated phenol solution at 50 °C, add other components and mix well. Solution is stored at 4 °C protected from light, and melted in a water bath at 50 °C then cooled to room temperature before use.

20. Phenol/chloroform/isoamyl alcohol (25:24:1) solution, pH 8.

21. 35 mg/ml glycogen.

22. 10 M ammonium acetate, pH 5.2.

23. 100 % ethanol.

24. 70 % ethanol.

25. Nuclease-free water.

26. Qubit broad-range dsDNA quantification assay (Invitrogen).

27. Drosophila 2× sonication buffer: 100 mM Tris–HCl pH 8, 20 mM EDTA, 2 % SDS. Buffer is made from stocks of individual components and stored at room temperature.

28. Bioruptor sonicator (Diagenode).

29. 3 M sodium acetate, pH 5.2.

2.2 Hi-C Method 1: Library Preparation and Sequencing

1. Nuclease-free water.

2. Repair mix (per reaction): 10 μl 10× T4 DNA ligase buffer (NEB), 4 μl 10 mM dNTPs mix, 5 μl (15 U) T4 DNA polymerase (NEB), 1 μl (5 U) DNA Polymerase I large (Klenow) fragment (NEB), 5 μl (50 U) T4 polynucleotide kinase (NEB). Mix is made fresh from individual components just before use and kept on ice.

3. QiaQuick PCR purification kit (Qiagen).

4. Adenylation mix (per reaction): 5 μl 10× NEB2 buffer (NEB), 10 μl 1 mM dATP, 3 μl (15 U) Klenow fragment (3′–5′ exo$^-$) (NEB). Mix is made fresh from individual components just before use and kept on ice.

5. MinElute PCR purification kit (Qiagen).

6. Adapter ligation mix (per reaction): 25 μl 2× DNA ligase buffer (Illumina), 10 μl PE adapter oligo mix (Illumina 1001782), 5 μl DNA ligase (Illumina). Mix is made fresh from individual components just before use and kept on ice.

7. Orange G loading dye.

8. SYBR Green I nucleic acid gel stain (Invitrogen).

9. Dark Reader Transilluminator (Clare Chemical).

10. QiaQuick gel extraction kit (Qiagen).

11. Phusion PCR mix (per reaction): 13 μl nuclease-free water, 25 μl 2× Phusion DNA polymerase mix (Illumina), 1 μl PCR primer PE 1.0 (Illumina 1001783), 1 μl PCR primer PE 2.0 (Illumina 1001784). Mix is made on ice from individual components just before use.

12. PCR thermal cycler.

13. Agilent 2100 Bioanalyzer with DNA 1000 reagents and chips.

2.3 Hi-C Method 2: Biotin-Mediated Purification of 3C Ligation Products in Mouse Hepatocytes

1. Scalpel.

2. 100 mm Petri dish.

3. PBS [Ca/Mg −/−].

4. 10 ml syringe.

5. 15 ml glass Dounce homogenizer with loose and tight pestles.

6. 70 μm cell strainer.

7. Trypan Blue.

8. Hemocytometer.

9. Mouse fixation buffer: 1× DMEM/F12 (Invitrogen), 1 % formaldehyde, 750 μg/ml bovine serum albumin (BSA) fraction V, 1 % penicillin/streptomycin (*see* **Note 1**).

10. Flatbed rocker.

11. 1 M glycine, room temperature.

12. Lysis buffer: 10 mM Tris–HCl pH 8, 10 mM NaCl, 0.2 % NP-40, EDTA-free protease inhibitor cocktail (Roche). Buffer is made fresh on the day of use and stored on ice.

13. 1× NEB2 buffer. Buffer is made from 10× stock from NEB (*see* **Note 2**).

14. Protein LoBind microcentrifuge tubes (Eppendorf; *see* **Note 4**).

15. 20 % SDS.

16. 20 % Triton-X100.

17. High-concentration HindIII (100,000 U/ml; NEB) (*see* **Note 2**).

18. Fill-in reaction buffer: 1× NEB2 buffer, 15 μM dATP, 15 μM dTTP, 15 μM dGTP, 15 μM biotin-14-dCTP, 125 U/ml DNA Polymerase I large (Klenow) fragment (NEB). Buffer is made fresh from stocks of individual components.

19. 1× T4 DNA ligase buffer (made fresh on day of use from 10× stock from NEB).

20. High-concentration T4 DNA ligase (2,000,000 U/ml; NEB).

21. 1× TE buffer: 10 mM Tris–HCl pH 8, 1 mM EDTA pH 8.

22. 10 mg/ml proteinase K stable at 65 °C (Bioline).

23. 20 mg/ml RNase A.

24. Phenol/chloroform/isoamyl alcohol (25:24:1) solution, pH 8.

25. Chloroform.

26. GlycoBlue (Ambion).

27. 3 M sodium acetate, pH 5.2.

28. 100 % ethanol.

29. 70 % ethanol.

30. Nuclease-free water.

31. BSA, molecular biology grade (NEB).

32. Qubit high-sensitivity (HS) and broad-range (BR) dsDNA quantification assay (Invitrogen).

33. NheI (10,000 U/ml; NEB)

34. T4 DNA polymerase (3000 U/ml; NEB).

35. Biotin removal buffer: 5 U T4 DNA polymerase, 100 μg/ml BSA, 100 μM dATP, and 100 μM dGTP in 100 μl 1× NEB2 buffer. This is the final composition of buffer for one reaction. As the volume of input DNA may vary, the reaction mixture is made fresh on the day of the experiment from individual components.

36. 0.5 M EDTA pH 8.0.

37. 1× TLE buffer: 10 mM Tris–HCl pH 8, 0.1 mM EDTA pH 8.

38. Covaris S220 focused ultra-sonicator.

2.4 Hi-C Method 2: Library Preparation and Sequencing

1. Fragment end repair buffer: 1× T4 DNA ligase buffer, 250 μM dNTP mix, 90 U/ml T4 DNA polymerase (NEB), 300 U/ml T4 polynucleotide kinase (NEB), 30 U/ml DNA polymerase I large (Klenow) fragment (NEB). Buffer is made fresh from stocks of individual components.

2. MinElute PCR Purification Kit (Qiagen).

3. 1× TLE buffer: 10 mM Tris–HCl pH 8, 0.1 mM EDTA pH 8.

4. Orange G loading dye.

5. SYBR Green I nucleic acid gel stain (Invitrogen).

6. Dark Reader Transilluminator (Clare Chemical).

7. QiaQuick Gel Extraction Kit (Qiagen).

8. Qubit high-sensitivity (HS) dsDNA quantification assay (Invitrogen).

9. Dynabeads MyOne Streptavidin C1 beads (Invitrogen) and magnet.

10. 1× Tween buffer: 5 mM Tris–HCl pH 8, 500 µM EDTA pH 8, 1 M NaCl, 0.05 % (v/v) Tween 20.

11. Rotating wheel.

12. 1× binding buffer: 5 mM Tris–HCl pH 8, 500 µM EDTA pH 8, 1 M NaCl.

13. 1× NEB2 buffer. Buffer is made from 10× stock from NEB.

14. Overhang buffer: 0.5× NEB2 buffer, 100 µM dATP, 50 U/ml Klenow fragment (3′–5′ exo⁻) (NEB). Buffer is made fresh from stocks of individual components.

15. 1× T4 DNA ligase buffer (made fresh on day of use from 10× stock from NEB).

16. PE adapters oligo mix (Illumina).

17. High-concentration T4 DNA ligase (2,000,000 U/ml; NEB).

18. Sequencing primers PE 1.0 and PE 2.0 (Illumina).

19. Herculase II Fusion polymerase kit (Agilent).

20. PCR thermal cycler.

21. AMPure beads

22. Agilent 2100 Bioanalyzer with DNA 1000 reagents and chips.

3   Methods

3.1   Hi-C Method 1: Direct Sequencing of 3C Material in Drosophila Embryos

The method described here is specific to Drosophila embryos. Other 3C protocols (e.g., [3]) that result in efficient digestion and re-ligation of chromatin in different tissues, including human samples, should be compatible with this method. The only specific need of this technique is that the digestion is performed with a frequently cutting restriction enzyme with a four base pair recognition motif. To perform this Hi-C approach on human samples, obtain the pure 3C DNA by alternative approaches (e.g., as for the "3C" tube in Section 3.3), but replacing the restriction enzyme and corresponding buffer with one cutting at four base pair motifs, then proceed with the technique from **step 25**. The efficiency of digestion and ligation by this different technique can be assessed as described below.

1. Transfer flies to embryo collection cages with egg-laying medium plates coated with yeast and set up laying schedules at 25 °C. For example, to collect 16–18 h embryos, add a fresh plate to the collection system at 25 °C and leave for 2 h; exchange for a fresh plate and incubate the old plate at 25 °C for a further 16 h.

2. Wash embryos from plate to collection sieve system in embryo collection buffer.

3. Dechorionate embryos by treating with bleach for 5 min.

4. Wash the embryos in distilled water and transfer ~3000 embryos (*see* **Note 5**) to a 50 ml falcon tube in embryo collection buffer.

5. Centrifuge at 2000 × g, 3 min, 4 °C and remove supernatant.

6. Resuspend embryos in 5 ml Drosophila fixation buffer (*see* **Note 1**) and dounce in Toenbroeck douncer. Transfer to 15 ml falcon tube and fix for a total time of 10 min (from addition of fixation buffer to quenching with glycine) at 25 °C with shaking at 750 rpm.

7. Quench with 5 ml 2 M glycine and put on ice.

8. Centrifuge at 4500 × g, 5 min, 4 °C, remove supernatant, and resuspend in 5 ml Drosophila wash buffer.

9. Centrifuge at 4500 × g, 5 min, 4 °C, remove supernatant, and resuspend in 5 ml 1.25× NEB3 buffer.

10. Centrifuge at 4500 × g, 5 min, 4 °C, remove supernatant, resuspend in 1 ml 1.25× DpnII buffer, and transfer nuclei to 1.5 ml microcentrifuge tube (*see* **Note 6**).

11. Centrifuge at 18,000 × g, 1 min, 4 °C, remove supernatant, and resuspend in 300 μl 1.25× DpnII buffer (*see* **Note 2**).

12. Add 7.5 μl 20 % SDS and incubate for 1 h at 37 °C, 750 rpm (*see* **Note 7**).

13. Add 34 μl 20 % Triton-X100 and incubate for 1 h at 37 °C, 750 rpm (*see* **Note 7**).

14. Add 30 μl (1500 U) DpnII and incubate overnight at 37 °C, 750 rpm (*see* **Notes 2** and **3**).

15. Add 26 μl 20 % SDS and incubate for 20 min at 65 °C, 750 rpm. For assessment of digestion efficiency, *see* **Notes 8** and **9** and Fig. 1a.

16. Transfer the chromatin to a 50 ml falcon tube containing 10 ml Drosophila ligation buffer and incubate for 1 h at 37 °C, 750 rpm.

17. Add 20 μl (40,000 U) T4 DNA ligase and incubate for 4 h at 25 °C, 750 rpm.

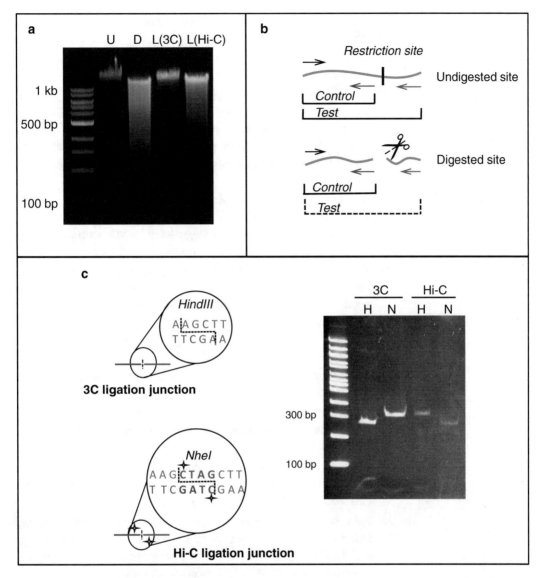

Fig. 1 Assessing the quality of a Hi-C library preparation. (**a**) 1 % agarose gel showing purified DNA from various stages of a Hi-C preparation, performed as in Section 3.3 on mouse hepatocytes. *U* undigested, *D* digested, *L(3C)* re-ligation (3C control), *L(Hi-C)* re-ligation (Hi-C template). Successful digestion and re-ligation is indicated by the shifts in gel mobility of the different samples. Note that when a four-cutter restriction enzyme is used (as in Section 3.1), the digested smear is expected to be for smaller DNA (densest staining at ~500–1000 bp). (**b**) A schematic of the qPCR strategy used to confirm successful digestion of 3C restriction sites. Primers are designed to either span the site (*black* and *red arrows*, "test amplification") or to a genomic site which does not contain a restriction site (*black* and *blue arrows*, "control amplification"). The control primer set will amplify both digested and undigested samples, while the test primer set will amplify only if the site has not been digested (here the *dashed line* indicates that the amplification has not occurred). The ratio of the products between the two primer sets is used to estimate the digestion efficiency at that particular site. Multiple sites in the genome can be analyzed in this way. (**c**) Schematic for Hi-C (Section 3.3), showing the ligation junction without (conventional 3C) or with (Hi-C) a successful filling-in reaction, and a 6 % gel showing comparative HindIII (H) and NheI (N) digests of a specific PCR product generated from 3C and Hi-C templates. *Crosses* represent biotinylated nucleotides which are found only at Hi-C ligation junctions

18. Add 75 μl 10 mg/ml proteinase K and incubate overnight at 65 °C, 750 rpm.

19. Cool to room temperature, add 40 μl 20 mg/ml RNase A and incubate for 1 h at 37 °C, 750 rpm.

20. Add 35 ml room temperature undersaturated phenol solution, mix vigorously by vortexing, and centrifuge at 7500 × g, 15 min, 25 °C (*see* **Note 10**). Transfer 1 ml of upper aqueous layer plus residual organic phase to microcentrifuge tube. Mix vigorously by vortexing and centrifuge at 18,000 × g, 4 min, room temperature.

21. Transfer upper aqueous phase to fresh microcentrifuge tube(s) in 400 μl batches (*see* **Note 10**). Add 400 μl phenol/chloroform/isoamyl alcohol, mix vigorously by vortexing, and centrifuge at 18,000 × g, 4 min, room temperature.

22. Transfer upper aqueous phase to fresh microcentrifuge tube and add 1 μl 35 mg/ml glycogen, 40 μl 10 M ammonium acetate, and 1 ml ethanol. Mix vigorously by vortexing and centrifuge at 18,000 × g, 40 min, 4 °C.

23. Remove supernatant and wash DNA pellet in 500 μl 70 % ethanol. Centrifuge at 18,000 × g, 5 min, 4 °C. Remove supernatant and dissolve DNA pellet in 50 μl nuclease-free water.

24. Quantify the 3C DNA with the Qubit broad-range dsDNA quantification assay, following the manufacturers' instructions (*see* **Notes 8** and **11**).

25. In a microcentrifuge tube on ice, mix 25 μl 3C DNA with 25 μl 2× Drosophila sonication buffer. Sonicate for three cycles (30 s on/30 s off; high power) with the Bioruptor.

26. Add 50 μl nuclease-free water, 100 μl phenol/chloroform/isoamyl alcohol and mix vigorously by vortexing. Centrifuge at 18,000 × g, 4 min, room temperature and transfer upper, aqueous phase to fresh microcentrifuge tube.

27. Add 1 μl 35 mg/ml glycogen, 10 μl 3 M sodium acetate, and 250 μl ethanol. Mix vigorously by vortexing and centrifuge at 18,000 × g, 40 min, 4 °C.

28. Remove supernatant and wash DNA pellet in 300 μl 70 % ethanol. Centrifuge at 18,000 × g, 5 min, 4 °C, remove supernatant and dissolve pellet in 20 μl nuclease-free water.

29. Quantify the DNA with the Qubit broad-range dsDNA quantification assay, following the manufacturers' instructions, and test sonication efficiency by loading a 500 ng aliquot on a 1 % agarose gel (*see* **Note 12**). Use 500 ng aliquots of 3C material for library preparation and sequencing (Section 3.2).

3.2 Hi-C Method 1: Library Preparation and Sequencing

This method describes the preparation of libraries compatible for paired-end Illumina sequencing from sonicated 3C DNA fragments. Overall, library preparation encompasses repair of DNA ends, then addition of an adenyl group at the 3′ end for subsequent ligation with paired-end adapter. These products are size-selected on agarose gels and then subjected to amplification with a limited number of PCR cycles. The library is tested for quality and then sequenced. The whole protocol essentially follows Illumina's guidelines, except that larger products are selected (*see* **Note 12**).

1. Make 500 ng aliquots of 3C DNA up to 75 μl with nuclease-free water. Add 25 μl repair mix and incubate for 30 min at 20 °C.

2. Purify the DNA with a QiaQuick PCR purification kit, following the manufacturers' instructions and eluting in 32 μl provided elution buffer.

3. Add 18 μl adenylation mix and incubate for 30 min at 37 °C.

4. Purify the DNA with a MinElute PCR purification kit, following the manufacturers' instructions and eluting in 10 μl provided elution buffer.

5. Add 40 μl adapter ligation mix and incubate for 15 min at 20 °C.

6. Purify the DNA with a MinElute PCR purification kit, following the manufacturers' instructions and eluting in 30 μl provided elution buffer.

7. Add Orange G loading buffer to the samples and run on a 1.5 % agarose gel, stain the gel with SYBR Green I (1× final concentration) for 30 min at room temperature, and visualize the DNA with a Dark Reader Transilluminator. Excise fragments of the appropriate size (*see* **Note 13**) and purify with a QiaQuick Gel Extraction kit, following the manufacturers' instructions and eluting each column in 30 μl provided elution buffer.

8. Set up PCR reactions by mixing 10 μl gel-extracted product aliquots with 40 μl Phusion PCR mix in PCR tubes on ice and run the following PCR reaction: 98 °C for 30 s (98 °C for 40 s, 65 °C for 30 s, 72 °C for 30 s) × 8–12 cycles (*see* **Note 14**), 72 °C for 5 min.

9. Pool PCR products originating from reactions using the same sample for the same number of PCR cycles and purify with a MinElute PCR purification kit, following the manufacturers' instructions and eluting in 30 μl provided elution buffer.

10. Quantify and obtain the size of the product by running 1 μl on an Agilent 2100 Bioanalyzer using a DNA 1000 assay, following the manufacturers' instructions (*see* **Note 14**).

11. Perform paired-end sequencing runs.

3.3 Hi-C Method 2: Biotin-Mediated Purification of 3C Ligation Products in Primary Mouse Hepatocytes

The Hi-C method described here is similar to the one first defined by Lieberman-Aiden [5], except for some minor modifications. We adapted the method for use with primary tissue samples and we routinely perform the ligation reaction in intact nuclei instead of in diluted conditions as per the original procedure. Our protocol involves multiple quality control steps to assess the efficiency of the digestion, ligation, and fill-in reactions.

1. Working on ice, use a scalpel to cut up the liver in small pieces on a 100 mm dish with PBS, then dissociate further using the sterile end of a 10 ml syringe.

2. Transfer the liver to a 15 ml glass Dounce homogenizer in 10 ml of PBS.

3. Homogenize ~10 times with the lower gauge pestle.

4. Top up the volume to 15 ml with PBS.

5. Homogenize ~10 times with the higher gauge pestle.

6. Filter the homogenized liver through a 70 μm cell strainer in a 50 ml falcon tube and top up the volume to 50 ml with PBS.

7. Centrifuge at $1230 \times g$, 5 min, 4 °C and remove supernatant.

8. Wash with 50 ml PBS, centrifuge at $1230 \times g$, 5 min, 4 °C, and resuspend in 15 ml PBS.

9. Dilute 5 μl of the cell resuspension with 15 μl Trypan Blue and load on a hemocytometer. Count the cells.

10. Aliquot the cells in universal tubes containing ~5×10^7 cells each and centrifuge at $1230 \times g$, 5 min, 4 °C. Remove the supernatant.

11. Resuspend each aliquot in 20 ml mouse fixation buffer and incubate at room temperature on a flatbed rocker for 10–30 min (*see* **Note 1**).

12. Quench the reaction by adding 2.5 ml of 1 M glycine (final concentration 125 mM). The medium will turn bright yellow.

13. Wash twice with cold PBS, centrifuging at $1230 \times g$, 5 min, 4 °C.

14. Aliquot 1×10^7 nuclei in universal tubes and pellet by centrifuging at $1230 \times g$, 5 min, 4 °C (*see* **Note 6**).

15. Resuspend cells in 10 ml lysis buffer and put on ice for 30 min.

16. Centrifuge at $1200 \times g$, 5 min, 4 °C and discard supernatant.

17. Resuspend nuclei in 1 ml 1× NEB2 buffer and transfer them to LoBind microcentrifuge tubes (*see* **Notes 2** and **4**).

18. Quick-spin the sample for 15 s at 4 °C, discard the supernatant, and resuspend the nuclei in 500 μl 1× NEB2 buffer (*see* **Note 2**).

19. Add 2.5 μl 20 % SDS and incubate for 1 h at 37 °C, 800 rpm (*see* **Note 7**).

20. Add 16.7 µl 20 % Triton-X100 and incubate for 1 h at 37 °C, 800 rpm (*see* **Note 7**).

21. Add 15 µl (1500 U) HindIII and incubate overnight at 37 °C, 800 rpm (*see* **Note 2**).

22. Add 5 µl (500 U) fresh HindIII and incubate for a further 3 h at 37 °C, 800 rpm (*see* **Note 2**).

23. Transfer 270 µl of the reaction mixture to a new microcentrifuge tube for the filling-in reaction (the "Hi-C" tube). The remaining reaction mixture (the "3C" tube) is processed as a normal 3C to allow assessment of the filling-in efficiency. Quick-spin each tube for 15 s at room temperature, discard supernatant, and resuspend in 1 ml 1× NEB2 buffer to wash away residual HindIII. For assessment of digestion efficiency, *see* **Notes 8** and **9** and Fig. 1a.

24. Quick-spin the "Hi-C" tube for 15 s at room temperature. Discard the supernatant and resuspend nuclei in 200 µl fill-in reaction buffer. Incubate at 37 °C for 45 min without shaking, but with mixing by inversion every 15 min (*see* **Note 15**).

25. Wash both the "3C" and "Hi-C" tubes twice in 100 µl 1× T4 DNA ligase buffer by quick centrifugation for 15 s at room temperature, discarding the supernatant and resuspending the nuclei in fresh buffer.

26. Quick-spin both the "3C" and "Hi-C" tubes for 15 s at room temperature. Discard the supernatant and resuspend nuclei in 100 µl 1× T4 DNA ligase buffer plus 2000 U T4 DNA ligase. Incubate overnight at 16 °C without shaking.

27. Add 300 µl 1× TE buffer and 40 µl 10 mg/ml proteinase K which is stable at 65 °C. Incubate overnight at 65 °C.

28. Cool to room temperature, add 10 µl 20 mg/ml RNase A, and incubate for 1 h at 37 °C.

29. Add 400 µl phenol/chloroform/isoamyl alcohol, mix vigorously by vortexing, and centrifuge at $18,000 \times g$, 5 min, room temperature.

30. Transfer upper aqueous phase to fresh microcentrifuge tube and add 400 µl chloroform. Mix vigorously by vortexing and centrifuge at $18,000 \times g$, 5 min, room temperature.

31. Transfer upper aqueous phase to fresh microcentrifuge tube and add 1 µl GlycoBlue, 40 µl 3 M sodium acetate, and 1.2 ml ethanol. Mix vigorously by vortexing and incubate for 1 h at −80 °C or overnight at −20 °C.

32. Centrifuge at $18,000 \times g$, 30 min, 4 °C. Remove supernatant, wash pellet in 500 µl 70 % ethanol, and centrifuge at $18,000 \times g$, 5 min, room temperature.

33. Remove supernatant and dissolve DNA pellet in 30 μl nuclease-free water.

34. Quantify the 3C and Hi-C DNA with the Qubit high-sensitivity (HS) dsDNA quantification assay, following the manufacturers' instructions. We have prepared a Hi-C library from as little as 10 μg of DNA (*see* **Note 11**).

35. Assess the fill-in efficiency (*see* **Note 16** and Fig. 1c). PCR-amplify a selection of ligation products from 25 ng of starting "3C" and "Hi-C" material in 50 μl reactions. Incubate 12.5 μl from each PCR amplification with HindIII (100 U) and 12.5 μl with NheI (100 U) overnight at 37 °C, then load the digestion reactions on precast vertical 6 % agarose TBE gels. Stain the gels by soaking them for 30 min in TBE containing 200 ng/ml ethidium bromide on a flatbed rocker, protected from light. Visualize the results under UV light.

36. Split the Hi-C DNA into 5 μg aliquots and make each aliquot into 100 μl reaction volumes of 1× biotin removal buffer. Incubate for 2 h at 12 °C (*see* **Note 17**).

37. Quench each reaction with 2 μl 0.5 M EDTA (pH 8), pool them together, and purify the DNA by phenol/chloroform extraction and ethanol precipitation (*see* **steps 30–33**). Dissolve the DNA in 100 μl TLE buffer.

38. Quantify the DNA with the Qubit broad-range dsDNA quantification assay, following the manufacturers' instructions (*see* **Note 11**).

39. Split the Hi-C DNA into 4 μg aliquots and make up each aliquot to a final volume of 120 μl in TLE buffer. Sonicate with the Covaris S220 focused ultra-sonicator, following the manufacturers' instructions and using these parameters: 20 % Duty Cycle, 5 Intensity, 200 cycles/burst, 140 s (*see* **Note 18**). Proceed with Section 3.4.

3.4 Hi-C Method 2: Library Preparation and Sequencing

This method varies from the library preparation in Section 3.2 by incorporating pull-down of the biotinylated 3C ligation junctions with streptavidin beads. Buffer exchange by washing the beads removes the need for multiple purification column steps.

1. Add 168 μl fragment end repair buffer to each aliquot and incubate for 30 min at 22 °C.

2. Purify the repaired DNA with the MinElute PCR purification kit, following the manufacturers' instructions. Use one column per aliquot and elute each in 30 μl TLE buffer.

3. Add Orange G loading buffer to the samples and run on a 1.5 % agarose gel, stain the gel with SYBR Green I (1× final concentration) for 30 min at room temperature, and visualize the DNA with a Dark Reader Transilluminator. Excise fragments

of the appropriate size (*see* **Note 13**) and purify with a QiaQuick Gel Extraction kit, following the manufacturers' instructions and eluting each column in 18 μl TLE.

4. Pool the aliquots and quantify the DNA with the Qubit high-sensitivity (HS) dsDNA quantification assay.

5. Wash Dynabeads MyOne Streptavidin C1 beads twice by resuspending in 400 μl Tween buffer and incubating for 3 min on a rotating wheel at room temperature, then removing the supernatant after putting the tubes on a magnet. Use 50 μl of beads per 2.5 μg Hi-C DNA.

6. Incubate the beads with the Hi-C DNA template in 360 μl binding buffer for 1 h on a rotating wheel at room temperature.

7. Wash the beads twice with 400 μl binding buffer and once with 400 μl 1× NEB2, each time incubating for 3 min on a rotating wheel at room temperature and discarding the supernatant after placing the tubes on the magnet.

8. Resuspend beads in 100 μl overhang buffer and incubate for 45 min at 37 °C.

9. Remove the supernatant after placing the tubes on a magnet and wash beads twice with 100 μl binding buffer and once with 100 μl T4 DNA ligase buffer, each time incubating for 3 min on a rotating wheel at room temperature and discarding the supernatant after placing the tubes on the magnet.

10. Resuspend washed beads in 1× T4 DNA ligase buffer plus 6 pmol Illumina paired-end adapters per μg of DNA, and add 1200 U T4 DNA ligase. Incubate ligation reaction overnight on a rotating wheel at room temperature.

11. Wash beads twice with 200 μl Tween buffer, four times with 200 μl binding buffer, and twice with 200 μl 1× NEB2 buffer, each time incubating for 3 min on a rotating wheel at room temperature, then removing the supernatant on a magnet. Resuspend beads in 50 μl 1× NEB2 buffer.

12. Set up 50 μl PCR reactions with 10 μl 5× Herculase II reaction buffer per 10 μl of beads, 2.5 μl DMSO, 1 μl 2.5 μM primer PE 1.0, 1 μl 2.5 μM primer PE 2.0, and 1 μl Herculase II Fusion polymerase. Run the following PCR reaction: 98 °C for 2 min (98 °C for 20 s, 65 °C for 30 s, 72 °C for 30 s) × 8–12 cycles (*see* **Note 14**), 72 °C for 5 min.

13. Purify the PCR product using AMPure beads, following the manufacturers' instructions.

14. Quantify and obtain the size of the product by running 1 μl on an Agilent 2100 Bioanalyzer using a DNA 1000 assay, following the manufacturers' instructions (*see* **Note 14**).

15. Pool PCR products originating from reactions using the same sample for the same number of PCR cycles.

16. Perform paired-end sequencing runs.

3.5 Hi-C Data Processing and Normalization

The process starts from the fastq files that are generated during Illumina Hi-Seq sequencing runs. After initial alignments, the kept paired reads are converted from coordinate space to restriction fragment end (fend) space. In 3C-based experiments the maximum theoretical resolution is at the level of the component restriction fragments that the genome is cut into. Thus, we consider interactions as pairwise combinations of the ends of these restriction fragments, rather than their exact genomic coordinates (Fig. 2a). A matrix of "observed counts" is all detected pairwise interactions from the Hi-C library and is normalized to the "expected" numbers of reads based on a model accounting for technical biases in the experiment [12]. The log-ratios of observed and expected reads for different genomic window sizes are plotted as the resultant Hi-C heatmap.

1. Align the fastq reads to the reference genome with the Bowtie software [13]. Discard all reads that do not uniquely map to a single genomic locus and perform the alignment for each half of a paired-end read separately (*see* **Note 19**).

2. From the output aligned reads, mate the aligned pairs. For each aligned "left" read, search for a corresponding "right" read with the same unique tag ID. Keep the appropriately mated aligned pairs and discard all reads with no corresponding mate.

3. From the reference genome, obtain the restriction map and define the fend table. Record all the genomic coordinates of recognition motifs for the restriction enzyme used in the Hi-C experiment to obtain a list of restriction fragments, recording each fragment's length in base pairs. For each restriction site, record the two fends on either side, recording its genomic coordinate, strand, and corresponding restriction fragment and fragment length (*see* Fig. 2a).

4. For each fend, determine its mappability (*see* **Note 20**). To obtain a genome-wide score of mappability, convert the reference genome into 50 bp fragments, overlapping each fragment by 10 bp (i.e., so that all nucleotides but for chromosome extremities are covered by five of these in silico fragments). Align these fragments back to the reference genome with Bowtie, keeping only uniquely mapping fragments. For each nucleotide in the genome, its mappability score is given by the number of these uniquely mapping fragments which cover the nucleotide, thus scoring from 0 (no mappability) to 5 (completely unique mappability). Determine the mean mappability score for the 500 bp terminal sequence of each fend

(or the entire restriction fragment, if it is shorter than 500 bp), convert this into a proportion of the maximal score (i.e., 5 = 100 % mappability), and discard fends with a mappability lower than the threshold (nominally 50 %; *see* **Note 21**). For the accepted mappability scores, stratify them into five equal-sized bins (e.g., bin 1 = 0.5–0.6, bin 5 = 0.9–1), and record these binned scores for each of the kept fends.

5. For each fend, also record the proportion of G and C nucleotides in the sequence, for the terminal 200 bp of the fend (or the total restriction fragment, if it is shorter).

6. Convert the united paired sequence reads into pairwise combinations of their corresponding kept fends, based on their mapped genomic coordinates. At this stage, self-ligation events or non-informative reads, where both reads map to the same restriction fragment, are discarded. These are particularly populous within Hi-C experiments where ligation products have not been preselected (Section 3.1).

7. Pairs where one or both of the ends correspond exactly to a restriction site are discarded. These reads comprise around 5–10 % of those from Hi-C experiments using restriction enzymes with a 4 bp recognition motif (*see* Section 3.1) and represent incomplete ligation events at the sequenced fragment termini, which seem to add noise to the data.

8. For Hi-C experiments without preselection of ligation junctions (*see* Section 3.1), plot a graph of frequency of read pairs against the distance in base pairs between the two ends. Make this plot for the four different combinations of strand orientations within the pairs (i.e., convergent or facing reads, divergent reads, and parallel reads facing "left" or "right"). For the facing reads, a local maximum of the population is expected at a size around ~600–800 bp, corresponding to the exact size selection in **step** 7 of Section 3.2. Discard facing/convergent reads with a separation smaller than this "facing threshold," as these are more likely to be undigested contiguous genomic fragments rather than genuine 3C ligation events (*see* Fig. 2b and **Note 22**).

9. From the fend table, stratify the GC proportions and fragment lengths into 20 bins of equal population (i.e., if there are 2000 fends in the fend table, set the value delimiters so that each bin contains 100 fends), each (1 = lowest, 20 = highest), and attribute a GC bin and a fragment length bin to each fend.

10. For all possible pairwise combinations of fends from different chromosomes (*see* **Note 23**), tally the occurrence of each combination of GC and fragment length bin (e.g., GC bin 1/fragment length bin 1 fend interacting with GC bin 1/fragment length bin 1 fend; GC bin 1/fragment length bin 1 fend

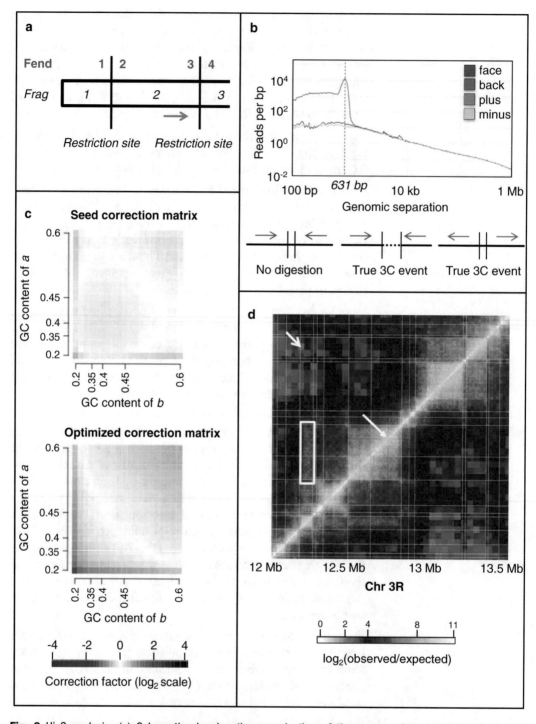

Fig. 2 Hi-C analysis. (**a**) Schematic showing the organization of the genome into restriction fragments (numbered in *black*) and their fragment ends (fends, numbered in *red*). The attribution of a mapped Hi-C sequence read to a fend depends on its corresponding fragment and read direction. In the example shown, the sequence read (*blue arrow*) corresponds to fend 3 (it would correspond to fend 2 if it was facing the opposite direction and thus restriction site). (**b**) Facing threshold analysis. Graph of frequency of read pairs from a Hi-C experiment using the four-cutter DpnII against the genomic separation between the two reads, stratified by the

interacting with GC bin 1/fragment length 2 fend, etc.). This represents the naïve expected proportions of interacting fends with different GC and fragment length characteristics.

11. Repeat **step 10** but for the kept observed Hi-C pairs output at **steps** 7 and **8**. This represents the actual observed proportion of interacting fends with different GC and fragment length characteristics.

12. Obtain the trans prior probability, Pr, for observing a specific combination of two fends on different chromosomes within the Hi-C experiment. This prior probability is based on the assumption that all fend combinations are equally likely to be observed:

$$Pr = \frac{\text{total observed trans fend pairs}}{\text{total possible trans fend pairs}}$$

13. Obtain the independent seed correction matrices for the GC content and fragment length of interacting fends (*see* Fig. 2c). In other words, the inherent bias or discrepancy between the expected (**step 10**) and observed (**step 11**) proportions of interacting fends with different GC and fragment length characteristics is expressed as a technical correction factor, which will be later used to normalize the Hi-C maps. For each combination of fend a (fends with a specific GC or fragment length bin) with fend b (fends with a specific GC or fragment length bin), the correction probability, $P_{GC}(a,b)$ or $P_{len}(a,b)$, is

---

Fig. 2 (continued) orientation of the two reads. Divergent reads ("back"; *blue arrows* in schematic) can only result from digestion and re-ligation of the genome, so must represent true 3C events. Facing reads (*red arrows* in schematic) may represent true 3C reads (central schematic) or, for reads that have very small genomic separation, contiguous genomic sequence that was not digested during the experiment. The overrepresentation of facing reads compared to other types of reads suggests that the latter case is more prevalent over short genomic separation (631 bp in this experiment). Facing reads shorter than this "facing threshold" are thus removed from subsequent analyses. (**c**) Technical normalization of Hi-C data. The seed (*top*) and finally optimized (*bottom*) correction matrices for fend GC content in a Hi-C experiment using the four-cutter DpnII. Interacting fends of lower GC content tend to be overrepresented in the Hi-C dataset, generating positive correction factors in the seed matrix. However, due to the much stronger biases created by restriction fragment length, and a non-independent relationship between fend GC content and fragment length, the optimized correction matrix actually follows the opposite trend. (**d**) Visual representation of Hi-C data. A heat map showing the log-ratio of observed and expected Hi-C reads over a 1.5 Mb region in a Drosophila Hi-C experiment. Topological domains are demarcated by *gray lines*. Multiple bin sizes are plotted simultaneously, from 5 kb windows (e.g., the *filled arrow*) to 40 kb windows (e.g., the *open arrow*); the smallest bin size with a minimum number of observed reads (in this case, 30) is plotted to show the best "useful" resolution across multiple regions. Note also that the color scheme is nonlinear to give better contrast between different interacting regions. For example, the color scheme allows an inter-domain interaction (*orange-yellow* color, region highlighted in *white rectangle*) to be distinguished from adjacent weaker interactions (*red* color), which themselves can be distinguished from the background (*blue* color)

calculated from the observed number of trans reads corresponding to interactions between a and b, obs(a,b), the total possible number of trans fend combinations corresponding to interactions between a and b, total(a,b), and the trans prior probability, Pr:

$$P(a, b) = \left(\frac{\mathrm{obs}(a, b)}{\mathrm{total}(a, b)} \right) / \mathrm{Pr}$$

14. To account for cross-correlations of GC content and restriction fragment length (*see* **Note 24**), optimize these seed correction matrices to increase their log-likelihood, LL, which is calculated by:

$$\mathrm{LL} = \sum (\mathrm{obs}(a, b) \times \mathrm{Psum}) + (\mathrm{diff}(a, b) \times \log_2(1 - \mathrm{Pprod}))$$

where Psum is the sum of the logs of the corrected probabilities used in the model,

$$\mathrm{Psum} = \log_2 \mathrm{Pr} + \log_2 P_{\mathrm{GC}}(a, b) + \log_2 P_{\mathrm{len}}(a, b)$$

diff(a,b) is the number of unobserved reads that would correspond to an interaction between a and b,

$$\mathrm{diff}(a, b) = \mathrm{total}(a, b) - \mathrm{obs}(a, b)$$

and Pprod is the product of the logs of the corrected probabilities used in the model,

$$\mathrm{Pprod} = \mathrm{Pr} \times P_{\mathrm{GC}}(a, b) \times P_{\mathrm{len}}(a, b)$$

Use the BFGS optimization method available in the R package maxLik [14] to optimize first the GC correction matrix, and then the fragment length matrix, recalculating the log-likelihood each time and continuing the optimization iterations until the log-likelihood difference between two iterations is less than 1.

15. If mappability is included in the model, the correction matrix is not optimized, but is a simple multiplicative probability of the mappability scores. For example, the correction factor for the interaction between a fend of mappability bin 1 (mappability score of 0.5–0.6) and a fend of mappability bin 3 (mappability score of 0.7–0.8) = $0.55 \times 0.75 = 0.4125$.

16. Based on the trans prior probability, Pr, and the final correction matrices, F_{GC}, F_{len} and F_{map}, the expected read count of any fend pair combination, $P(X_{a,b})$, can now be expressed as:

$$P(X_{a,b}) = \mathrm{Pr} \times F_{\mathrm{GC}}(a_{\mathrm{GC}}, b_{\mathrm{GC}}) \times F_{\mathrm{len}}(a_{\mathrm{len}}, b_{\mathrm{len}}) \\ \times F_{\mathrm{map}}(a_{\mathrm{map}}, b_{\mathrm{map}})$$

In other words, the expected probability is the trans prior probability multiplied by the appropriate correction factors for the component fends' GC proportions, fragment lengths, and mappabilities. The mappability correction term is simply excluded if it is not being used in the modeling, such as for *Drosophila melanogaster*. Split the genome into fixed-size bins (e.g., 100 kb; *see* **Note 25**). For each pairwise bin combination, sum the observed Hi-C counts and sum the expected counts for all possible fend combinations that correspond to the genomic bin combination. The Hi-C interaction score is expressed as log2(observed/expected) and can be plotted as a heat map to derive the final Hi-C interaction map (*see* **Note 26** and Fig. 2d).

4   Notes

1. The fixation buffer should be prepared fresh every time a new batch of cells is cross-linked. The formaldehyde in the fixation buffer is diluted from a 37 % (w/v) formaldehyde saturated aqueous solution, called "formalin." It is important to note that the concentrations reported in this method are formaldehyde percentages, not formalin percentages (e.g., a 1 % formaldehyde solution would be a 2.7 % formalin solution). When dissolved in water, formaldehyde exists mostly as monomers of methylene glycol. With time, these molecules have a strong tendency to spontaneously polymerize and can be oxidized to formic acid when the solution comes into contact with air. Methanol (10–15 %) is added to formalin as a stabilizer, as it can inhibit both of these reactions. There is no consensus on how long formalin should be stored, but it is advisable to use small bottles that can be used over a short amount of time, so as to minimize the decay of the reagent owing to repeated contact with air and/or methanol/formaldehyde evaporation. The optimal formaldehyde concentrations and fixation times can vary with tissue type. When starting a Hi-C experiment in a new cell or tissue type, it is advisable to run controls to check the efficiency of digestion and ligation (*see* **Notes 8** and **9**). If digestion is inefficient, the formaldehyde concentration or fixation time may need to be decreased.

2. These described protocols use DpnII (Section 3.1) or HindIII (Section 3.3) as the 3C restriction enzyme, but other enzymes can be chosen depending on the distribution of their restriction sites within the genome of the organism used in the experiment. Be sure to replace the described restriction buffers with those that are compatible with the chosen enzyme. Note also that many restriction enzymes are not suitable for Hi-C due to their inefficiency at digesting cross-linked chromatin. Test the digestion efficiency of new enzymes (*see* **Notes 8** and **9**) before

scaling up to full Hi-C experiments. Enzymes which have been shown to work in 3C experiments include BglII [15], NcoI [5] and EcoRI [2] (six-cutters), and NlaIII [11] (although this enzyme needs to be stored at −80 °C) and Csp6I [16] (four-cutters).

3. For Section 3.1, it is crucial to use a frequently cutting enzyme with a 4 bp recognition motif. If the enzyme cuts too sparsely within the genome, very few of the finally sequenced products will contain ligation junctions and thus be informative about genomic interactions.

4. Some cell or nuclei preparations can be very sticky, so LoBind tubes are recommended to prevent loss of material during buffer exchanges.

5. Using too many Drosophila embryos in one Hi-C batch affects the ligation efficiency. If available, the best way of counting dechorionated embryos is by large particle flow cytometry using a COPAS platform (Union Biometrica). Otherwise, test the ligation efficiencies (*see* **Note 8**) for different sizes of embryonic pellet derived at **step 5** of Section 3.1 to get a visual idea of the experiment limits.

6. Fixed nuclei (Section 3.1) or cells (Section 3.3) can be stored at this step. Remove the entire supernatant, flash freeze the pellet in liquid nitrogen, and store at −80 °C for up to a few months. When continuing with the experiment, thaw the pellet on ice for 30 min prior to resuspending in restriction buffer (Section 3.1) or lysis buffer (Section 3.3).

7. SDS incubation is required to solubilize the non-cross-linked proteins and to permeabilize the nuclei. The Triton-X100 is in turn used to quench the SDS by sequestering it in micelles. Conditions need to be adjusted for specific samples. For particularly problematic samples, it may be necessary to increase the SDS concentration to 0.6 % and/or incubate with SDS for 30 min at 65 °C and then move the samples to 37 °C for another 30 min. The amount of Triton-X100 added will depend on the amount of SDS to sequester: as a general rule, a 1 % final concentration of Triton-X100 is used to quench 0.3 % SDS.

8. Before investing resources into high-throughput sequencing, it is important to assess the quality of the 3C material. If specific chromatin loops are already known in the tissue being studied, recapitulation of these established results by qPCR (see [3] for experimental details) makes an ideal quality control. Whether or not this approach is feasible, it is also important to test that the digestion and ligation steps of the 3C experiment work efficiently. These can be qualitatively assessed by comparing the size profiles of the purified genomic DNA taken before

digestion, after digestion but before ligation, and after ligation. Take 20–30 μl aliquots of material just before digestion (Section 3.1, **step 13**; Section 3.3, **step 20**) and 20–30 μl aliquots of material just after digestion (Section 3.3. **step 15**; Section 3.3, **step 23**) and purify the DNA as for the rest of the Hi-C material (heat treatment with proteinase K to remove cross-links, RNase A treatment, phenol/chloroform/isoamyl alcohol extraction, ethanol precipitation, wash with 70 % ethanol, resuspension of DNA pellet in nuclease-free water, and quantification with a Qubit dsDNA assay). Load 500 ng–1 μg samples on a 1 % agarose gel, along with equal amounts of final 3C material (Section 3.1, **step 24**; Section 3.3, **step 34**). Undigested material should form a tight band with low mobility in the gel. The digested material should form a smear of much higher mobility, whose exact size profile will depend on the restriction site used (Fig. 1a). The re-ligated samples should have a much greater apparent size, ideally resembling the original undigested material. It should be noted that in Section 3.3, the "Hi-C" sample tends to have a lower ligation efficiency than the "3C" sample, presumably due to greater difficulty in ligating blunt ends and/or inefficiencies in the fill-in process (Fig. 1a).

9. Digestion efficiency can also be assessed quantitatively at a limited number of restriction sites by qPCR. For each restriction site to be tested, design three qPCR primers: a forward primer facing the tested site, and two complementary reverse primers, one within the same restriction fragment as the forward primer (forming an internal control product, C), and another on the other side of the tested site (forming the digestion test product, T; *see* Fig. 1b). Perform qPCR reactions on 20 ng template DNA taken from the same before/after digestion steps mentioned in Note 8. The digestion efficiency is inversely proportional to the amplification efficiency of the digestion test product, as digested molecules are not amplifiable. Thus, the digestion efficiency can be quantified as:

$$1 - \left(\frac{R_{\text{digested}}}{R_{\text{undigested}}} \right)$$

where

$$R = \frac{\text{amplification}_T}{\text{amplification}_C}$$

10. Using undersaturated (90 %) phenol at this step absorbs a lot of the water from the ligase buffer, resulting in a much smaller volume of aqueous solution which is more convenient for ethanol precipitation. If the solution stays transparent after mixing with the phenol, add 1 ml of nuclease-free water and

re-vortex; repeat until solution is no longer transparent. The subsequent extraction with phenol/chloroform/isoamyl alcohol is performed in 400 µl batches so that ethanol precipitation can be performed in 1.5 ml microcentrifuge tubes.

11. Due to the ATP and DTT which can be precipitated from the ligase buffer, standard A_{260} spectrophotometry measurements are unreliable for quantifying 3C material. It is much more accurate to use the Qubit system which measures the fluorescence of a dye which intercalates specifically with double-stranded DNA.

12. For Section 3.1, it is desirable to sequence products of size between 600 and 800 bp to maximize the chance of trapping an informative ligation junction. Some optimization of the sonication conditions may be required, depending on the sample, but all conditions will produce quite a broad smear of different-sized products.

13. The desired size of the products to be extracted from the gel depends on the initial Hi-C method used. For Section 3.2, the extraction is performed after adapters have been incorporated; a size of 700–900 bp is important (an insert size of 600–800 bp (*see* **Note 12**) plus ~100 bp for the incorporated adapter sequence). For Section 3.4, the gel extraction takes place before adapter incorporation, and a more conventional size of 150–300 bp is acceptable.

14. The PCR reaction is needed to add the sequencing primers to the fragments and to increase the library concentration before the last quality control. The number of PCR cycles at this stage should be kept to a minimum, though, as each round of amplification will decrease the complexity of the library. An advisable strategy is to run a first round of amplification on one aliquot of your library using a low number of cycles (as low as 8), purify and run the reaction product on the Bioanalyzer. If a profile is visible and gives a single peak, the rest of the sample can be amplified using the same number of cycles. Conversely, if a profile is not visible (below 4 ng/µl) or the sample looks too concentrated (more than 20 ng/µl), it is possible to raise or drop the number of cycles, respectively, for the rest of the library. If it is necessary to change the number of cycles, pool only the aliquots that were amplified with the "correct" amount of cycles. If peaks corresponding to unincorporated primers and/or primer dimers are detected, consider changing the primer concentrations in the PCR reaction or performing a gel extraction (Section 3.3, **step 3**) between the PCR and Bioanalyzer steps.

15. The Klenow DNA polymerase I fragment retains 5′–3′ exonuclease activity and can start to remove nucleotides from the

filled-in ends if kept at 37 °C too long. It is therefore important to not exceed the incubation time.

16. The fill-in of a digested HindIII site introduces a new cutting site for NheI and abolishes the original HindIII site in properly re-ligated fragments. Thus the 3C template ligation junctions should be cut by HindIII but not NheI, whereas the Hi-C template ligation junctions should be cut by NheI, but not HindIII. In order to assess the fill-in efficiency, a set of ligation junctions are amplified by PCR and the sensitivity to cutting by the two different restriction enzymes is assayed and visualized on a gel. The primers for ligation junction amplification can be designed flanking HindIII cutting sites at known interacting loci or, alternatively, flanking two randomly selected neighboring but nonadjacent HindIII cutting sites (i.e., cutting sites that are close to one another, but do not belong to the same fragment); these latter are expected to interact due to proximity. It is possible that not all ligation junctions in the cell population will have been filled in successfully, giving rise to the appearance of both undigested and digested bands on the gel. The efficiency of the fill-in at a certain site will be given by the ratio between the undigested band and the digested band(s) (*see* Fig. 1c).

17. The ends that have not been successfully re-ligated are not informative, but will still contain the biotin and thus could end up in the pool of fragments that will be sequenced in the Hi-C library. To prevent this, the biotin is removed from the unligated ends before pull-down with streptavidin. In order to do so, the sample is incubated with T4 DNA polymerase for 2 h to promote 3′–5′ digestion of the labeled 5′-AGCT-3′ in the unligated ends. The biotin is attached to the cytosine in this tetra-nucleotide. dATP and dGTP are added to the reaction to limit the spread of the exonuclease activity to the last two nucleotides of the unligated ends.

18. At this stage it is possible to check the size of the sheared DNA by running 1 μl of the sonicated material on an Agilent 2100 Bioanalyzer using a DNA 1000 assay, following the manufacturers' instructions. The size of the bulk of the fragments should be between 150 and 400 bp. Use of the Agilent 2100 Bioanalyzer to check DNA shearing in Section 3.1 is not more informative than running a gel, as the distribution of product sizes is broad.

19. To avoid any ambiguity in the interpretation of Hi-C interaction datasets, it is important to only keep uniquely aligning sequence tags. To ensure this in Bowtie, use the option −*m 1*. Default quality cut-off parameters (−*n 2 −e 70*; meaning a maximum of two mismatches are allowed, and a minimal

quality score of 70) usually work well, but can be altered for problematic genome alignments. Other high-performance alignment programs should work, but be sure to set the parameters to ensure that only uniquely mapping tags are kept, and take precautions that the quality scales for the program and the input fastq files are compatible.

20. This protocol normalizes the Hi-C interaction map for up to three technical parameters which are shown to cause over- or underrepresentation of certain sequences for nonbiological reasons: mappability, restriction fragment length, and local fragment end GC content [12]. As only uniquely aligned tags are kept in the analysis, restriction fragments containing completely unique sequence are more easily represented in the processed Hi-C data than those fragments containing fewer stretches of uniquely aligned sequence. Short restriction fragments tend to be underrepresented in Hi-C datasets, possibly due to torsional strains reducing their cohesive ends' mobility during ligation. Restriction fragment ends with a high local GC content are more difficult to melt during sequencing, and are thus underrepresented in Hi-C datasets.

21. In mammalian genomes, it is sensible to discard fends with mappability lower than 50 %, as these have so few uniquely aligning and thus usable sequence. Some genomes have very little variability in mappability—almost all of the *Drosophila melanogaster* genome is comprised of either unique sequence or highly repetitive sequence. In this case, it is more appropriate to discard all fends with less than 100 % mappability and to not incorporate mappability in the technical normalization.

22. Use the same facing threshold when comparing multiple Hi-C datasets. As the choice of facing threshold affects only the very short-range interactions, it is also possible to choose a conservative threshold a priori (e.g., 1 kb) and avoid generating the graphs at this step. However, these graphs are useful quality controls in their own right.

23. *Cis* interaction strengths are influenced heavily by the genomic separation between the interacting points [5, 7]. Restricting the modeling of technical features to interchromosomal interactions removes this confounding factor.

24. The correction matrices obtained in **step 13** correct for biases in the Hi-C data for restriction fragment length and GC content independently, but there may be cross-correlations between these factors (e.g., shorter fragments may have a different GC content profile to longer fragments). To prevent overcorrection for certain factors, the model needs to be optimized as in **step 14**. The differences between the seed and final correction matrices depend on the genome and restriction

enzyme used; for example, restriction fragment length tends to be a much more important factor for frequently cutting restriction enzymes.

25. The best bin width(s) to use depends on factors which affect the resolution of the interaction being studied: genome size, sequencing depth and, for *cis* interactions, the genomic separation of the interacting points. This last point is especially important, as different bin widths will be required to capture different scales of interactions within the same Hi-C experiment. For example, high resolution will be required to capture a specific short-range chromatin loop, but the same resolution will look like background noise at megabase-scale distances. A lower resolution/larger bin size may detect specific domain co-associations at megabase distance but will not resolve the short-range loops. One way to present the Hi-C data on the multiple scales required is to simultaneously plot the heat maps for multiple bin widths on top of each other, but to omit the plotting of higher-resolution maps for parts of the matrix where the sequence coverage is below a certain threshold (*see* Fig. 2d). Thus, the highest resolution that is reasonably likely to be informative is plotted throughout the heat map. The exact bin widths to use to best represent the Hi-C data need to be empirically determined for each experiment.

26. Similarly to the resolution discussed in Note 25, the interaction strength across a genome-wide map can vary by three orders of magnitude, especially when studying *cis* interactions. As well as using a log scale for the heat map, it is advisable to try different color schemes with nonlinear gradients between them, in order to obtain the greatest contrast between interacting regions and background over multiple distance scales (*see* Fig. 2d). Again, these color schemes need to be empirically determined from the data.

References

1. Lanctot C, Cheutin T, Cremer M et al (2007) Dynamic genome architecture in the nuclear space: regulation of gene expression in three dimensions. Nat Rev Genet 8:104–115

2. Dekker J, Rippe K, Dekker M et al (2002) Capturing chromosome conformation. Science 295:1306–1311

3. Thierry Forne's chapter in this same book…

4. Dekker J, Marti-Renom MA, Mirny LA (2013) Exploring the three-dimensional organization of genomes: interpreting chromatin interaction data. Nat Rev Genet 14:390–403

5. Lieberman-Aiden E, van Berkum NL, Williams L et al (2009) Comprehensive mapping of long-range interactions reveals folding principles of the human genome. Science 326:289–293

6. Dixon JR, Selvaraj S, Yue F et al (2012) Topological domains in mammalian genomes identified by analysis of chromatin interactions. Nature 485:376–380

7. Sexton T, Yaffe E, Kenigsberg E et al (2012) Three-dimensional folding and functional organization principles of the Drosophila genome. Cell 148:458–472

8. Seitan VC, Faure AJ, Zhan Y et al (2013) Cohesin-based chromatin interactions enable regulated gene expression within preexisting

architectural compartments. Genome Res 23:2066–2077

9. Sofueva S, Yaffe E, Chan WC et al (2013) Cohesin-mediated interactions organize chromosomal domain architecture. EMBO J 32:3119–3129

10. Zuin J, Dixon JR, van der Reijden MI et al (2014) Cohesin and CTCF differentially affect chromatin architecture and gene expression in human cells. Proc Natl Acad Sci U S A 111:996–1001

11. van de Werken HJ, Landan G, Holwerda SJ et al (2012) Robust 4C-seq data analysis to screen for regulatory DNA interactions. Nat Methods 9:969–972

12. Yaffe E, Tanay A (2011) Probabilistic modeling of Hi-C contact maps eliminates systematic biases to characterize global chromosomal architecture. Nat Genet 43:1059–1065

13. http://bowtie-bio.sourceforge.net/index.shtml

14. http://www.maxlik.org/

15. Schoenfelder S, Sexton T, Chakalova L et al (2010) Preferential associations between co-regulated genes reveal a transcriptional interactome in erythroid cells. Nat Genet 42:53–61

16. Raab JR, Chiu J, Zhu J et al (2012) Human tRNA genes function as chromatin insulators. EMBO J 31:330–350

Methods in Molecular Biology (2017) 1589: 75–88
DOI 10.1007/7651_2015_269
© Springer Science+Business Media New York 2015
Published online: 30 May 2016

Quantitative Analysis of Intra-chromosomal Contacts: The 3C-qPCR Method

Vuthy Ea, Franck Court, and Thierry Forné

Abstract

The chromosome conformation capture (3C) technique is fundamental to many population-based methods investigating chromatin dynamics and organization in eukaryotes. Here, we provide a modified quantitative 3C (3C-qPCR) protocol for improved quantitative analyses of intra-chromosomal contacts. We also describe an algorithm for data normalization which allows more accurate comparisons between contact profiles.

Keywords: Chromosome conformation capture, Chromatin dynamics and organization, Quantitative PCR

1 Introduction

During the last decade, the advent of the chromosome conformation capture (3C) technique [1] and derived technologies (4C, 5C ...) [2–4] has allowed researchers to explore the organization and the dynamics of the eukaryotic genomes with unprecedented resolution and accuracy. Recently, a new approach, combining the 3C technique with high-throughput sequencing (Hi-C method), provided the first glimpses on global chromatin architecture and dynamics in the yeast *Saccharomyces cerevisiae* [5], the fly *Drosophila melanogaster* [6], the mouse *Mus musculus domesticus* [7], and in the human [8]. The creation of a 3C library is therefore a prerequisite to many 3C-based methods. By freezing all chromatin contacts present at a given time in their physiological nuclear context, and then by averaging these events over a population of several millions of cells, the 3C-qPCR method [9] allows very accurate measurements of the relative interaction frequencies between chromatin segments, in *cis*, on the same chromosome (Fig. 1). This parameter is a key to investigate the in vivo dynamics of the chromatin because it depends not only on its fundamental biophysical parameters (compaction, rigidity ...) [10] but also on important locus-specific factors which are controlling local genomic functions (epigenetic modifications, binding of specific factors ...) [11]. Here we provide

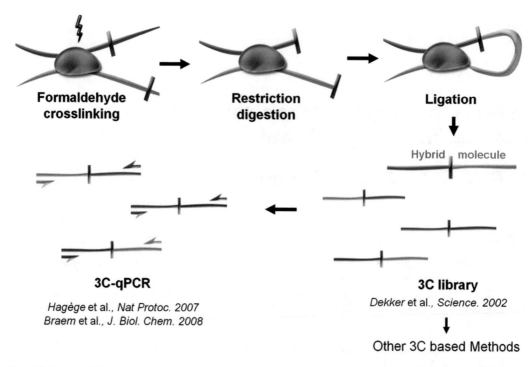

Fig. 1 Principle of the chromosome conformation capture (3C) assay. The principle of the 3C technique relies on three essential steps: formaldehyde cross-linking, restriction digestion, and ligation, providing a 3C library composed of hybrid DNA molecules. The relative interaction frequency of each ligated DNA fragment that reflects their physical proximity can be accurately determined by quantitative PCR (3C-qPCR method). The 3C library can also be used for other 3C-based methods, like the 4C, 5C, or Hi-C assays (see text for references)

a modified 3C-qPCR protocol that increases about fourfold the efficiency of the assay compared to the initial protocol [9]. We also describe an algorithm for very accurate normalizations 3C-qPCR data. Normalized data can then be more easily compared even if they come from very different biological samples [12].

2   Materials

2.1   Reagents and Biological Material

1. Tissues or cultured cells.

2. 10 % (v/v) FCS/PBS (catalog number D8537) (Sigma Chemical Company, St. Louis, MO, USA).

3. 40 μm cell strainer (catalog number 352340) (BD Falcon, Franklin Lakes, NJ, USA).

4. 37 % (v/v) formaldehyde (catalog number 47629) (Fluka, Sigma Chemical Company, St. Louis, MO, USA).

5. Glycine 1 M (catalog number 26-128-6405-C) (Euromedex, Souffelweyersheim, France).

6. 20 % w/v Sodium Dodecyl Sulfate (SDS) (catalog number EU0660) (Euromedex, Souffelweyersheim, France).

7. Triton X-100 (catalog number 2327140) (BDH Chemicals, Fontenay-sous-Bois, France).

8. 3C buffer (50 mM Tris–HCl pH 8.0; 50 mM NaCl; 10 mM MgCl$_2$; 1 mM dithiothreitol (DTT)).

9. High concentration Restriction Enzyme (40U/μl) (Fermentas, Burlington, Canada).

10. T4 DNA ligase high concentration (20U/μl) (Promega France, Charbonnières-les-Bains, France).

11. Ligation buffer (Fermentas, Burlington, Canada) (40 mM Tris–HCl pH 7.8; 10 mM DTT; 10 mM MgCl$_2$; 5 mM ATP).

12. ATP (catalog number R0441) (Fermentas, Burlington, Canada).

13. Ribonuclease A (RNase A) 1 mg/ml.

14. Proteinase K (PK) 10 mg/ml.

15. PK buffer (5 mM EDTA pH 8.0; 10 mM Tris–HCl pH 8.0; 0.5 % SDS).

16. UltraPure^{TM} buffer saturated Phenol (pH 7.5–7.8) (catalog number 15513-047) (Invitrogen, Carlsbad, NM, USA).

17. Chloroform (catalog number 438601) (Carlo Erba, Val-de-Reuil, France).

18. UltraPure^{TM} Phenol:Chloroform:Isoamyl alcohol 25:24:1 (v/v) (catalog number 15593-49) (Life Technologies, Carlsbad, CA, USA).

19. Anhydrous absolute ethanol (99.9 % v/v) (catalog number 414607) (Carlo Erba, Val-de-Reuil, France).

20. Oligonucleotide PCR primers, user specific (see Reagent setup). *GAPDH* primer sequences used for loading controls (Section 3.9, step 1) are as follows: forward primer: ACAGTC-CATGCCATCACTGCC, reverse primer: GCCTGCTTCACC ACCTTCTTG.

21. SYBR^{R} Green PCR Master Mix as described in ref. [13] with modifications described in refs. [10, 11] (also *see* Section 3.9, step 1).

22. Hot-Start Taq *Platinum* Polymerase (catalog number 10966-34) (Life Technologies, Carlsbad, CA, USA).

23. GoTaq G2 Hot Start (catalog number M740B) (Promega France, Charbonnières-les-Bains, France).

24. CleanAmp 3'THF dNTP (catalog number 040 N-9501-10) (Tebu-bio, Le Perray, France).

25. BAC (Invitrogen, Carlsbad, NM, USA).

26. Reagent setup: Primers used in quantitative PCR are typically 21–23 mers with a Tm in the range of 55–65 °C with a 2 °C maximum difference between primers used in one experiment. They should be designed close (50 bp) to the restriction site used for the 3C assays.

27. Prepare genomic DNA from the same organism as the samples to be investigated. Determine its concentration by O.D. measurements. This will constitute the genomic DNA of known concentration used in Section 3.9, step 1, for loading adjustment of samples.

28. Equipment setup: Microcentrifuge, for example Eppendorf 5415 D, rotor F45-24-11 (for 1.5 ml tubes).

29. Eppendorf centrifuge 5810R (for 15 and 50 ml Falcon tubes).

30. Orbital shaker (INFORS HT TR-225).

31. LightCycler 480 II apparatus (Roche, Basel, Switzerland) and LightCycler 480 Software, release 1.4.9.0803.

3 Methods

3.1 Cell Nucleus Preparation

1. – If working with tissues, prepare nuclei as previously described in refs. [14, 15] and proceed with Section 3.2, step 1, below.

   – If working with cultured cells proceed to step 2 in Section 3.1.

   – If working with adherent cell cultures trypsinize, wash, and filter through 40 μm cell strainer to make a single-cell suspension before proceeding with step 2 in Section 3.1.

2. Wash cells in PBS.

3. Resuspend cells in 1.5 ml buffer 1 (0.3 M sucrose; 60 mM KCl; 15 mM NaCl; 5 mM $MgCl_2$; 0.1 mM EGTA; 15 mM Tris–HCl pH 7.5; 0.5 mM DTT; 0.1 mM PMSF; 3.6 ng/ml aprotinin; 5 mM Na-butyrate).

4. Add 0.5 ml buffer 2 (composition: as buffer 1 + 0.8 % v/v NP40) and mix slightly.

5. Put on ice for 2 or 3 min.

6. Put 1 ml in 14 ml tubes (×2 tubes) containing 4 ml buffer 3 (buffer 3: 1.2 M sucrose; 60 mM KCl; 15 mM NaCl; 5 mM $MgCl_2$; 0.1 mM EGTA; 15 mM Tris–HCl pH 7.5; 0.5 mM DTT; 0.1 mM PMSF; 3.6 ng/ml aprotinin; 5 mM Na-butyrate). Save a 4 μl aliquot to count nuclei in a Thoma cell (this allows to determine nucleus concentration that will then be adjusted as explained in step 9 below).

7. Centrifuge for 20 min at 8500 rpm (11,300 × g) at 4 °C.

8. Remove supernatant (use several tips to avoid NP40 contamination of the nucleus pellet).

9. Resuspend pellets in glycerol buffer (40 % v/v glycerol; 50 mM Tris–HCl pH 8.3; 5 mM MgCl$_2$; 0.1 mM EDTA) to achieve a final concentration of about 20 million nuclei in 100 μl.

10. Freeze into liquid nitrogen and store at −80 °C.

3.2 Formaldehyde Cross-Linking

1. Take 5×10^6 nuclei and make up to 700 μl with 3C buffer (50 mM Tris–HCl pH 8.0; 10 mM MgCl$_2$; 50 mM NaCl; 1 mM DTT).

2. Carefully resuspend nuclei with the pipet and leave for 5 min at room temperature.

3. Add 19.7 μl of formaldehyde (final concentration 1 %), mix by tumbling the tube, and hold at room temperature for precisely 10 min.

4. Add 80 μl of 1.25 M glycine (125 mM final) to neutralize the formaldehyde. Mix by slowly tumbling the tube and wait precisely for 2 min at room temperature. Stop the reaction by putting the tube on ice for at least 5 min.

5. Centrifuge for 3 min at 2,300 × *g* at room temperature, and remove supernatant (SN). Carefully resuspend the pellet with the pipet by adding 1 ml of 3C buffer (50 mM Tris–HCl pH 8.0; 10 mM MgCl$_2$; 50 mM NaCl; 1 mM DTT) (*see* **Note 1**).

6. Centrifuge for 3 min at 2,300 × *g* at room temperature, and remove the supernatant (SN).

3.3 Restriction Digestion

1. Take up the nuclei in 0.1 ml of 3C buffer and transfer to a safe-lock tube.

2. Place the tube at 37 °C and add 1 μl 20 % (w/v) SDS (final: 0.2 % SDS).

3. Incubate at 37 °C for 35 min while shaking at 200 rpm and then 35 min more at 37 °C while shaking at 120 rpm.

4. Add 16.8 μl of 10 % (v/v) Triton X-100 diluted in ligation buffer (40 mM Tris–HCl pH 7.8; 10 mM MgCl$_2$; 10 mM DTT; 5 mM ATP). Mix by carefully pipetting up and down to resuspend any deposit that may form.

5. Incubate at 37 °C for 35 min while shaking at 200 rpm and then 35 min more at 37 °C while shaking at 120 rpm.

6. Take a 10 μl aliquot of the sample as the "undigested control" (do not disturb the mixture). This sample may be stored at −20 °C until it is needed to determine the digestion efficiency (*see* Section 3.4, steps 1–24).

7. Add 450 U of the selected restriction enzyme (e.g., HindIII) to the remaining sample and incubate overnight at 37 °C while shaking gently (at 120 rpm for the first 2 h, then at 200 rpm). Mix very carefully with the pipet tip when adding the enzyme (*see* **Note 2**).

8. Take a 10 μl aliquot of the sample as the "digested control" (do not disturb the mixture). To process the remaining sample, continue to step 1 in Section 3.5. To determine the digestion efficiency, analyze the control aliquots from step 6 to step 8 in Section 3.3 as described in Section 3.4, steps 1–24. This analysis can be carried out in parallel with steps 1–10 in Section 3.5 (*see* **Note 3**).

3.4 Determination of Digestion Efficiencies

Digestion efficiencies have a significant impact on the assays and should be carefully assessed for each restriction site involved in the analysis; a twofold drop in digestion efficiency of a given site causes a twofold reduction in the amount of available restriction ends, which would affect the number of ligation products that can be detected for this fragment. Therefore, care should be taken to ensure that digestion efficiencies are in the same range for the sites of interest.

1. Add 500 μl of PK buffer (5 mM EDTA pH 8.0; 10 mM Tris–HCl pH 8.0; 0.5 % SDS) and 1 μl of 20 mg/ml Proteinase K (20 μg final) to the aliquot saved in Section 3.3, steps 6/8.

2. Incubate for 30 min at 65 °C (or overnight at 65 °C if performed in parallel to step 10 in Section 3.5).

3. Equilibrate at 37 °C, then add 1 μl of 1 mg/ml RNase A (1 μg final), and incubate for 2 h at 37 °C.

4. Add 500 μl of phenol-chloroform-isoamyl alcohol 25:24:1 (v/v) and mix vigorously.

5. Centrifuge for 5 min at $16,100 \times g$ at room temperature.

6. Transfer the supernatant into a new tube and add 50 μL of 2 M sodium acetate pH 5.6, and then 1.5 ml of anhydrous absolute ethanol (99.9 % v/v).

7. Mix and place at −80 °C till frozen (about 45 min).

8. Centrifuge for 20 min at $16,100 \times g$ at 4 °C.

9. Remove the supernatant and add 500 μl of 70 % ethanol.

10. Centrifuge for 4 min at $16,100 \times g$ at room temperature.

11. Remove the supernatant and dry the pellet at room temperature.

12. Take up the DNA pellet in 500 μl of restriction buffer (commercial 10× buffer for StyI or any another selected restriction enzyme diluted at 1× with distilled water) (*see* **Note 4**).

13. Add 1 μl of 1 mg/ml RNase A (1 μg final).

14. Add 5 μl of 10 U/μl StyI enzyme (Eco130I) (Fermentas, Burlington, Canada) (50 U final).

15. Incubate for 2 h at 37 °C.

16. Add 500 μl of phenol-chloroform and mix vigorously.

17. Centrifuge for 5 min at 16,100 × g at room temperature.

18. Transfer the supernatant into a new tube and add 25 μl of 5 M NaCl, and then 1 ml of anhydrous absolute ethanol (99.9 % v/v).

19. Mix and store at −20 °C overnight.

20. Centrifuge for 20 min at 16,100 × g at 4 °C.

21. Remove the supernatant and add 200 μl 70 % ethanol.

22. Centrifuge for 4 min at 16,100 × g at room temperature.

23. Resuspend the pellet in 60 μl of water.

24. Perform real-time PCR quantification (Syb^{R}Green) (as explained in Section 3.10, step 1 below) on undigested genomic DNA (UND; taken from step 6 in Section 3.3) and digested material (D; taken from step 8 in Section 3.3). Use primer sets that amplify across each restriction site of interest (R). To correct for any difference in the amount of template added to the PCR reaction, also PCR amplify control regions (C) not containing the restriction sites of interest; see qPCR reaction conditions see below (Section 3.10, step 1). The restriction efficiency is calculated according to the following formula: % Restriction = $100 - 100 / 2 \wedge ((Ct_R - Ct_C)_D - (Ct_R - Ct_C)_{UND})$ (*see* **Note 5**).

3.5 Ligation

1. Add 12 μl of 20 % (v/v) SDS (final 1.6 %) to the remaining sample from step 8 in Section 3.3.

2. Incubate for 30 min at 37 °C while shaking gently (120 rpm).

3. Transfer with caution the digested nuclei to a 12 ml tube (Greiner) (*see* **Note 6**).

4. Add 3.28 ml ligation buffer.

5. Add 390 μl of 10 % (v/v) Triton X-100 diluted in ligation buffer (final 1 % Triton X-100).

6. Incubate for 2 h at 37 °C while shaking gently (200 rpm).

7. Centrifuge for 1 min at 2200 × g at 4 °C.

8. Put the tube on ice and remove 3.27 ml of supernatant to leave 500 μl in the tube.

9. Add 6.5 μl ligase HC 30 U/μl and add 3 μl ATP 100 mM to the remaining 500 μl. Mix carefully by pipetting up and down.

10. Incubate overnight at 16 °C.

3.6 DNA Purification

1. Add 2 ml of 2× PK buffer and 1.5 ml H_2O.
2. Add 5 µl of 20 mg/ml Proteinase K (100 µg final).
3. Incubate for 1 h at 50 °C.
4. Incubate for 4 h at 65 °C to de-cross-link the sample.
5. Incubate for 1 h at 37 °C.
6. Add 4 ml of phenol and mix vigorously.
7. Centrifuge for 15 min at 2200 × g at room temperature (*see* **Note 7**).
8. Transfer the supernatant into a new 12 ml tube and add 4 ml of chloroform. Mix vigorously.
9. Centrifuge for 15 min at 2200 × g at room temperature.
10. Transfer the supernatant into a new 12 ml tube and add 200 µl of 5 M NaCl, 1 µl glycogen, and then 8 ml of anhydrous absolute ethanol (99.9 % v/v).
11. Mix and place at −20 °C overnight.
12. Centrifuge for 45 min at 2200 × g at 4 °C.
13. Remove the supernatant and add 2 ml of 70 % ethanol.
14. Centrifuge for 15 min at 2200 × g at 4 °C.
15. Remove the supernatant and briefly dry the pellet at room temperature.

3.7 Complementary Digestion

1. Take up the DNA pellet in 500 µl of restriction buffer (commercial 10× buffer for StyI or any another selected restriction enzyme diluted at 1× into distilled water) (*see* **Note 8**).
2. Place the sample into a 1.5 ml tube and add 5 µl of 1 mg/ml RNase A (5 µg final).
3. Add 10 µl of 10 U/µl StyI enzyme (100 U final).
4. Incubate for 2 h 30 min at 37 °C.
5. Add 500 µl of phenol-chloroform and mix vigorously.
6. Centrifuge for 5 min at 16,100 × g at room temperature.
7. Transfer the supernatant into a new tube and add 25 µl of 5 M NaCl, and then 1 ml of anhydrous absolute ethanol (99.9 % v/v).
8. Mix and store at −20 °C overnight.
9. Centrifuge for 20 min at 16,100 × g at 4 °C.
10. Remove the supernatant and add 200 µl 70 % ethanol.
11. Centrifuge for 4 min at 16,100 × g at room temperature.
12. Remove the supernatant and dry the pellet at room temperature.
13. Resuspend the pellet in 150 µl of 10 mM Tris–HCl pH 7.5 (*see* **Note 9**).

3.8 Assessment of Sample Purity (Optional)

1. Dilute two aliquots of the 3C sample (from step 13 in Section 3.7) (one twofold and the other fourfold). Add genomic DNA to the diluted reaction samples such that the total DNA concentration in each reaction is constant and around 25 ng/μl.

2. Perform quantifications with any 3C primer pair (*see* Section 3.10, step 1) and check that real-time PCR quantifications are reduced according to the dilution factors. If this is not the case the sample purity is not adequate and the sample as prepared from step 13 in Section 3.7 should be either re-purified or discarded.

3.9 Performing Loading Adjustments

1. Determine the DNA concentration of the 3C sample relative to a reference sample of genomic DNA of known concentration (see regent setup in Section 2, step 27). This can be done by Syb^{R}Green quantitative PCR on dilutions of 3C samples and the reference sample, using "internal" primer sets that do not amplify across sites recognized by any of the restriction enzymes used (e.g., *GAPDH* gene primers). Reaction conditions are as follows (10 μl final reaction volume): 1 μl of sample, 7 μl of H_2O, 1 μl of primer pair (5 μM each), and 1 μl of qPCR mix [for a detailed composition of the qPCR mix *see* ref. [13]. PCR parameters used for programming the thermal cycler (LightCycler, Roche) are as follows: 1 cycle: 3 min at 95 °C; 45 cycles: 1 s at 95 °C/5 s at 60 °C/15 s at 72 °C. Denaturation curve: 1 cycle: 45 °C: 30 s and then increase the temperature to 95 °C at a rate of 0.2 °C/s (*see* **Note 10**).

2. Adjust the original 3C samples (from step 13 in Section 3.7) with H_2O to approximately 25 ng/μl +/−10 % and, for each sample, determine again this concentration precisely by repeating the measurements as described in Section 3.9, step 1. These last values will be used later as "loading controls" of the samples (*see* Section 3.12, step 1).

3.10 Real-Time PCR Quantifications of Ligation Products

1. Perform real-time PCR quantifications to obtain the Ct of each ligation products on 1 μl (containing ~25 ng of DNA) of the "adjusted" 3C samples (from step 2 in Section 3.9). Reaction conditions are as follows (10 μl final reaction volume): 2 μl of sample, 1 μl of primer pair (5 μM each), 1 μl of qPCR mix, and 6 μl of H_2O. 3C products can be quantified using a LightCycler 480 II (Roche, Basel, Switzerland) (10 min at 95 °C followed by 45 cycles of 10 s at 95 °C/8 s at 69 °C/14 s at 72 °C) using the Hot-Start Taq *Platinum* Polymerase (Life Technologies, Carlsbad, CA, USA) or the GoTaq G2 Hot Start (Promega France, Charbonnières-les-Bains, France) and a standard 10× qPCR mix [13] where the usual 300 μM dNTP has been replaced by 1500 μM of CleanAmp 3'THF dNTP (*see* **Note 11**).

3.11 PCR Control Template Used for Primer Efficiency Control

1. A control template containing all ligation products in equal amounts is used to optimize real-time quantitative PCR (qPCR) reactions and to establish the minimal amount of ligation product that can still be quantified in a reliable manner. For this qPCR control template, we recommend the use of a single BAC clone covering the genome segment under study. Alternatively, a set of minimally overlapping BAC clones mixed in equimolar amounts can be used. This BAC is then cut with the restriction enzyme of choice (e.g., HindIII) and religated by T4 DNA ligase. A secondary restriction enzyme (e.g., StyI) can be used to linearize DNA circles which may otherwise affect primer hybridization efficiency [16]. It is then necessary to make serial dilutions of this reaction to obtain standard curves which cover the same range of ligation product concentrations as those that will be obtained in the 3C samples. To mimic 3C sample conditions, the final DNA concentration in these dilutions is adjusted to the amount of DNA used in the 3C samples (~25 ng/μl, see above Section 3.9, steps 1 and 2). Thus, these dilutions are performed in a 25 ng/μl DNA solution made of genomic DNA digested with the second restriction enzyme (e.g., StyI in the present protocol). Using serial dilutions of this control template, a standard curve with specific parameters (slope and intercept) is thus obtained for each of the 3C-qPCR primer pairs used. These parameters will be used below (Section 3.12, step 1) to correct for potential differences in primer efficiencies.

3.12 3C-qPCR Data Normalization: Primer Efficiency and Loading Controls

1. To obtain quantification values that are corrected for potential differences in primer efficiencies, the Ct obtained for each chimerical ligation product (Section 3.10, step 1) are first normalized using the parameters of the corresponding standard curve (the slope "a" and the intercept "b" obtained in Section 3.11, step 1). These values are calculated using the following formula: Value $= 10^{(Ct-b)/a}$. For each sample, these values are then normalized to the corresponding "loading control" obtained in Section 3.9, step 2 (make a ratio).

3.13 3C-qPCR Data Normalization: Normalization to Noise Band

The following normalization compensates for experimental variations and allows comparison between different 3C assays (*see* ref. [12]); it replaces *Pdhb* or *Ercc3* normalizations frequently used (*see* ref. [9]). The procedure below (Sections 3.13.1–3.13.3) should be followed independently for each sample. It is used for experiments designed to determine contact frequencies between a fixed ("constant" or "anchor") site and other sites spread *in cis* throughout the same genomic region (*see* **Note 12**).

3.13.1 Removal of "Deviant" Experimental Points

1. Removal can only be done when at least three independent 3C assays have been performed for a given sample. When only one or two independent assays have been performed, select all points and go to step 1 in Section 3.13.2 of the procedure.

2. For each experimental point (from step 1 in Section 3.12), calculate the Log of the values "v" normalized to *Gapdh* (Normalization 1) [Log v].

3. For each fragment (fx), calculate the mean [m(fx)] of [Log v].

4. For each fragment (fx), calculate the standard error of the mean [sem(fx)] of [Log v].

5. For each experimental point corresponding to a given fragment (fx), calculate $x(fx) = m(fx) - (sem(fx) \times k)$, where "k" is the "tolerance factor" that we usually fix at 1.05 (*see* **Note 13**).

6. For each experimental point corresponding to a given fragment (fx), calculate $y(fx) = m(fx) + (sem(fx) \times k)$, where "k" is the "tolerance factor" that we usually fix at 1.05 (*see* **Note 13**).

7. For each fragment (fx), select all experimental points for which $x(fx) < [Log\ v] < y(fx)$ and discard all other points.

3.13.2 Determination of the Basal Interaction Level

1. For each experimental point selected above (Section 3.13.1, step 7) corresponding to a given fragment (fx), calculate the mean of values "v" normalized to Gapdh (Section 3.12, step 1) [m'(fx)].

2. For each experimental point selected above (Section 3.13.1, step 7) corresponding to a given fragment (fx), calculate the standard error of the mean of the values normalized to Gapdh "v" (Section 3.12, step 1) [sem'(f)].

3. Calculate the mean [M] of all the [m'(fx)] values.

4. Calculate the mean [SEM] of all [sem'(fx)] values.

5. For each fragment (fx), select all experimental points for which $m'(fx) < M - (SEM)$.

6. Calculate the mean [M1] of all the [m'(fx)] values of the points selected in Section 3.13.2, step 5.

7. Calculate the standard error of the mean [SEM1] of all the [m'(fx)] values of the points selected in Section 3.13.2, step 5.

8. For each fragment (fx) amongst experimental points selected in Section 3.13.1, step 7, select experimental points for which $m'(fx) > M1 - (SEM1)$.

9. Calculate the mean [M2] of all the [m'(fx)] values of the points selected in Section 3.13.2, step 8.

10. Calculate the standard error of the mean [SEM2] of all the [m'(fx)] values of the points selected in Section 3.13.2, step 8.

11. The value of M2 is the "raw basal interaction level" (BIL) that we then use to normalize our data (*see* Section 3.13.3, step 1, below); M2 +/− SEM2 is the "raw noise band."

3.13.3 Normalization to the BIL and Determination of the Noise Band

1. For each fragment (fx), calculate the normalized mean M(fx) = m'(fx)/M2.

2. For each fragment (fx), calculate the normalized standard error of the mean SEM(fx) = sem'(fx) / M2.

3. Calculate the normalized BIL = M2/M2 = 1.

4. Calculate the normalized noise band NB = SEM2/M2.

5. BIL +/− NB is the "normalized noise band."

6. Make a graph showing the distribution of the M(fx) values ("relative cross-linking frequencies") as a function of the distance (in kb) between the fx fragments and the "constant/anchor" fragment.

4 Notes

1. Rinse the walls of the tube that have been in contact with the reaction mixture.

2. For better digestion efficiencies, the 450 U of enzyme may be added sequentially: first add 150 U and incubate for 2 h at 37 °C shaking at 120 rpm, then add 150 U and incubate for 2 h at 37 °C shaking at 200 rpm, and finally add 150 U and incubate overnight at 37 °C while shaking at 120 rpm. When using an enzyme other than HindIII adjust buffer composition as appropriate.

3. The percentage of digestion should be at least 60 %, but preferably >80 %. When using an enzyme other than HindIII, check that the composition of the recommended restriction buffer is not too different from the 3C buffer used in the present protocol.

4. Check that the corresponding restriction site (StyI in the present protocol) is absent from the PCR amplicons used to assess digestion efficiencies.

5. The efficiency of the restriction enzyme digestion should be above 60–70 %, but ideally >80 % is digested. Samples with lower digestion efficiencies should be discarded.

6. If the aqueous phase is very turbid after the first extraction, repeat the phenol extraction a second time.

7. Do not rinse the wall of the tube.

8. Check that the corresponding restriction site (StyI in the present protocol) is absent from the PCR amplicons used for ligation product quantification.

9. If some precipitates do not resuspend, dissolve DNA by gently shaking tubes at 37 °C for up to 30 min. The 3C template may be kept at −20 °C for several months.

10. Optical density (OD_{260}) measurements fail to provide an accurate estimate of DNA concentration in 3C samples, probably because of their limited purity. If qPCR reactions are performed in a different thermocycler (than the LightCycler, Roche) the PCR parameters may need to be optimized.

11. Do not use the CleanAmp dNTP 3'TBE (catalog number 040 N-9506) (Tebu-bio, Le Perray, France).

12. Note that this normalization procedure requires performing quantifications of interaction frequencies between each chosen "anchor site" and several "negative control sites," where no "specific/functional" interactions are expected, inside the same genomic region of interest. Such "negative control sites" should be located at least 35 kb from the "anchor site." These are necessary to calculate the BIL specific to each genomic region investigated. The BIL is then used to normalize the interaction profiles.

13. The "tolerance factor" (k) can be adjusted, depending on the goals of the experiment, to increase or decrease the threshold used to identify and remove the "deviant" experimental points.

Acknowledgement

This work was supported by grants from the *Institut National du Cancer* [contract N° INCa_5960, PLBIO 2012-129, to T.F.], the *Association pour la Recherche contre le Cancer* [ARC contract n°SFI20101201555 to T.F.], the *Ligue contre le cancer* (comité Hérault), and the *Centre National de la Recherche Scientifique* (CNRS).

References

1. Dekker J, Rippe K, Dekker M, Kleckner N (2002) Capturing chromosome conformation. Science 295:1306–1311

2. Dostie J, Richmond TA, Arnaout RA, Selzer RR, Lee WL, Honan TA, Rubio ED, Krumm A, Lamb J, Nusbaum C, Green RD, Dekker J (2006) Chromosome Conformation Capture Carbon Copy (5C): a massively parallel solution for mapping interactions between genomic elements. Genome Res 16:1299–1309

3. Simonis M, Klous P, Splinter E, Moshkin Y, Willemsen R, de Wit E, van Steensel B, de Laat W (2006) Nuclear organization of active and inactive chromatin domains uncovered by chromosome conformation capture-on-chip (4C). Nat Genet 38:1348–1354

4. Zhao Z, Tavoosidana G, Sjolinder M, Gondor A, Mariano P, Wang S, Kanduri C, Lezcano M, Sandhu KS, Singh U, Pant V, Tiwari V, Kurukuti S, Ohlsson R (2006) Circular

chromosome conformation capture (4C) uncovers extensive networks of epigenetically regulated intra- and interchromosomal interactions. Nat Genet 38:1341–1347

5. Duan Z, Andronescu M, Schutz K, McIlwain S, Kim YJ, Lee C, Shendure J, Fields S, Blau CA, Noble WS (2010) A three-dimensional model of the yeast genome. Nature 465:363–367

6. Sexton T, Yaffe E, Kenigsberg E, Bantignies F, Leblanc B, Hoichman M, Parrinello H, Tanay A, Cavalli G (2012) Three-dimensional folding and functional organization principles of the Drosophila genome. Cell 148:458–472

7. Dixon JR, Selvaraj S, Yue F, Kim A, Li Y, Shen Y, Hu M, Liu JS, Ren B (2012) Topological domains in mammalian genomes identified by analysis of chromatin interactions. Nature 485:376–380

8. Lieberman-Aiden E, van Berkum NL, Williams L, Imakaev M, Ragoczy T, Telling A, Amit I, Lajoie BR, Sabo PJ, Dorschner MO, Sandstrom R, Bernstein B, Bender MA, Groudine M, Gnirke A, Stamatoyannopoulos J, Mirny LA, Lander ES, Dekker J (2009) Comprehensive mapping of long-range interactions reveals folding principles of the human genome. Science 326:289–293

9. Hagège H, Klous P, Braem C, Splinter E, Dekker J, Cathala G, de Laat W, Forné T (2007) Quantitative analysis of chromosome conformation capture assays (3C-qPCR). Nat Protoc 2:1722–1733

10. Court F, Miro J, Braem C, Lelay-Taha M-N, Brisebarre A, Atger F, Gostan T, Weber M, Cathala G, Forné T (2011) Modulated contact frequencies at gene-rich loci support a statistical helix model for mammalian chromatin organization. Genome Biol 12:R42

11. Court F, Baniol M, Hagège H, Petit JS, Lelay-Taha M-N, Carbonell F, Weber M, Cathala G, Forné T (2011) Long-range chromatin interactions at the mouse Igf2/H19 locus reveal a novel paternally expressed long non-coding RNA. Nucleic Acids Res 39:5893–5906

12. Braem C, Recolin B, Rancourt RC, Angiolini C, Barthes P, Branchu P, Court F, Cathala G, Ferguson-Smith AC, Forné T (2008) Genomic matrix attachment region and chromosome conformation capture quantitative real time PCR assays identify novel putative regulatory elements at the imprinted Dlk1/Gtl2 locus. J Biol Chem 283:18612–18620

13. Lutfalla G, Uzé G (2006) Performing quantitative reverse-transcribed polymerase chain reaction experiments. Methods Enzymol 410:386–400

14. Milligan L, Antoine E, Bisbal C, Weber M, Brunel C, Forné T, Cathala G (2000) H19 gene expression is up-regulated exclusively by stabilization of the RNA during muscle cell differentiation. Oncogene 19:5810–5816

15. Milligan L, Forné T, Antoine E, Weber M, Hemonnot B, Dandolo L, Brunel C, Cathala G (2002) Turnover of primary transcripts is a major step in the regulation of mouse H19 gene expression. EMBO Rep 3:774–779

16. Weber M, Hagège H, Lutfalla G, Dandolo L, Brunel C, Cathala G, Forné T (2003) A real-time polymerase chain reaction assay for quantification of allele ratios and correction of amplification bias. Anal Biochem 320:252–258

Methods in Molecular Biology (2017) 1589: 89–98
DOI 10.1007/7651_2015_268
© Springer Science+Business Media New York 2015
Published online: 01 July 2016

5-Hydroxymethylcytosine Profiling in Human DNA

John P. Thomson, Colm E. Nestor, and Richard R. Meehan

Abstract

Since its "re-discovery" in 2009, there has been significant interest in defining the genome-wide distribution of DNA marked by 5-hydroxymethylation at cytosine bases (5hmC). In recent years, technological advances have resulted in a multitude of unique strategies to map 5hmC across the human genome. Here we discuss the wide range of approaches available to map this modification and describe in detail the affinity based methods which result in the enrichment of 5hmC marked DNA for downstream analysis.

Keywords: 5-hydroxymethylcytosine, 5hmC, 5mC, DNA immunoprecipitation and enrichment, HmeDIP, Epigenetics

1 Introduction

In the past few years there have been a host of studies investigating the modified base 5-hydroxymethylcytosine (5hmC) as well as the dioxygenase enzymes (the 10–11 translocation proteins 1-3 or TET1-3) responsible for the generation of this mark from a 5mC precursor [1–4]. Interestingly, although 5hmC is invoked as an intermediate in active DNA demethylation pathways it has also been found to reproducibly map to particular genomic loci suggesting it can be relatively stable and have a distinct function independent of DNA demethylation [2, 3, 5, 6]. Initial studies investigating 5hmC levels were primarily antibody based. Antibodies specific to 5hmC were used to both immuno-quantify global levels of 5hmC (a technique called "dot blotting" similar in principle to Western blotting) and to profile 5hmC genome-wide using an approach similar to the widely used technique of methyl DNA immunoprecipitation (MeDIP) [7]. Dot blotting has since been carried out on a host of human tissue types and has given relative values that are in agreement with biochemical measurements [8, 9]. Such studies revealed that global levels of 5hmc varied greatly between tissues types, while 5mC levels were relatively stable [9]. 5hmC antibody-based affinity techniques have in turn been described as hydroxymethyl-DNA immunoprecipitation or "Hme-DIP" and used to investigate the genome wide patterns of 5hmC in both cell lines as well as tissues. These studies in combination with downstream bioinformatic analysis have revealed that the majority of 5hmC is found in the genic portions of the genome in a transcriptional dependant manner, as well as at enhancer elements and promoter proximal regions (for a review see [2]. The potential for 5hmC profiling for diagnostic purposes has been described [10, 11] with particular focus placed on the progression of cancer in which the global levels of 5hmC are often found to be dramatically reduced [12].

Subsequently, alternative methods have been developed to enrich for 5hmC marked DNA, all of which are based on the ability to specifically discriminate between 5hmC and 5mC. Early work found that bisulfite conversion, a widely used method of 5mC analysis (bisulfite sequencing), was unable to discriminate between 5mC and 5hmC modified CpGs upon direct sequencing of converted substrates [13]. However, sodium bisulfite treatment does convert 5hmC into cytosine-5-methylenesulfonate (CMS), which can subsequently be immunoprecipitated using a highly specific antiserum to the CMS modification [14]. Although the CMS antibody appears to be highly specific, this approach relies heavily on the overall efficiency of conversion into CMS making it less attractive than HmeDIP.

Antibody independent methods of 5hmC enrichment have also been developed which are ultimately based on the ability of T4 phage enzyme beta-gylucosyltransferase (βGT) to specifically target 5hmC modified cytosines for glycosylation. Treatment with βGT alongside specially modified versions of dUTP nucleotides (i.e., containing a biotin group) effectively sugar coat the 5hmC portions of the genome resulting in a template for enrichment either by biotin/streptavidin (hydroxymethyl selective chemical labelling; "hMeSeal") or specific protein affinity (through the use of the trypanosome J binding protein 1; "JBP-1 affinity") based purification strategies [15–17]. The former of these two approaches has since been used extensively to map the 5hmC modification in a host of human and mouse tissues and cell lines [17–20]; however, these require either the use of commercially available kits, which can be prone to batch variation of enzymatic activity, or extensive chemical synthesis of the components required for purification. Aside from affinity based enrichment strategies, it is possible to study both the 5hmC and 5mC patterns at a single base resolution (by either oxidative bisulfite sequencing; "OxBS-seq" or TET assisted bisulfite sequencing; "TAB-seq") [21, 22]. Although ultimately such approaches will yield the most accurate picture of the epigenetic landscape, it is predicted that around $100\times$ coverage of the genome is required in order to confidently quantify the levels of DNA modification present at a given CpG, making such approaches incredibly expensive [23].

On balance, the antibody based hydroxymethyl-DNA immunoprecipitation (HmeDIP) approach remains one of the most routinely used methods for 5hmC enrichment. Most downstream analysis involves the use of tiling arrays in hybridization studies or next-generation sequencing of 5hmC enriched fractions to determine its profile in the analyzed sample [10]. Alternative 5hmC assay methods have been used to validate 5hmC profiling studies [24]. The fact that the HmeDIP protocol does not require the use of any particularly specialized pieces of equipment, as well as the ability to return DNA fragments which are widely used in many types of downstream application, means that it is one of the more popular routes of 5hmC enrichment. In short this approach relies on the relative ability to return 5hmC marked portions of the genome from a small percentage of the input and can be broken down into five main sections (Fig. 1): (1) The fragmentation of the DNA to a mean size of 500 bp through sonication, (2) incubation of fragmented DNA with an antibody specific to 5hmC, (3) incubation with beads which specifically bind to antibody bound fragments, (4) washing of the beads to remove nonspecific binding, and (5) the release of 5hmC enriched fragments. The immunoprecipitated DNA can then be compared to control DNA which was not subjected to immunoprecipitation (input) for a host of downstream applications such as qPCR analysis of candidate loci, hybridization to tiling microarrays, or next-generation sequencing.

2   Materials

Use analytical grade RNase/Dnase-free water was throughout. All solutions are to be stored at 4 °C unless stated otherwise.

2.1   Solutions and Reagents

1. IP Buffer (10×): 100 mM Na-Phosphate pH 7.0 (mono-dibasic), 1.4 M NaCl, 0.5 % Triton X-100. For 10 mL add 2 mL 0.5 M Na-Phosphate pH 7.0 (mono-dibasic), 2.8 mL 5 M NaCl, 0.5 mL 10 % Triton X-100, and 4.7 mL H_2O. Store at 4 °C.

2. Digestion Buffer (1×): 50 mM Tris pH 8.0, 10 mM EDTA, 0.5 % SDS. For 10 mL add 0.5 mL 1 M Tris pH 8.0, 0.2 mL 0.5 M EDTA, 0.25 mL 20 % SDS and 9.05 mL H_2O. Store at 4 °C.

3. 0.5 M Potassium phosphate bibasic and monobasic: For 100 mL, add 21.1 mL 1 M Potassium Phosphate Monobasic, 28.9 mL 1 M Potassium Phosphate Dibasic and 50 mL H_2O.

4. PBS-BSA (0.1 %): For 10 mL add 1 mL of 10 mg/mL Bovine Serum Albumin (BSA) and 9 mL Phosphate Buffered Saline (PBS).

5. TE: 10 mM Tris pH 8.0, 1 mM EDTA. For 10 mL add 0.1 mL of 1 M Tris–HCl (pH 8.0) and 0.02 mL EDTA (0.5 M) and 9.88 mL H_2O.

6. 5-hydroxymethylcytosine (5hmC) antibody (pAb) (ActiveMotif, CA, USA).

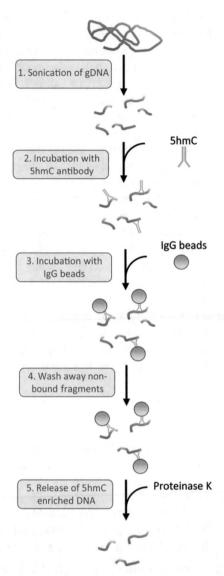

Fig. 1 An overview of the key stages in the HmeDIP protocol. (1) Genomic DNA is sheared to a mean size of 500 bp using a sonicator device (we recommend the use of the Diagenode Bioruptor®, Diagenode®, NJ, USA). (2) The small fragments of DNA are then incubated alongside the 5hmC antibody which will bind to CpGs modified by the 5hmC mark. (3) Following antibody binding, magnetic IgG beads are added which bind to the 5hmC antibody. Following binding, fragments of DNA lacking the 5hmC mark are removed by a series of washes (4). The remaining DNA fragments can finally be released from the IgG beads by proteinase K digestion of the associated antibodies (5)

7. [Optional] 5hmC-spike in control DNA (New England Bio-labs, CA, USA or Zymo Research, CA, USA).

8. Dynabeads protein G (Life Technologies, Paisley, UK).

9. Proteinase K dissolved in water to 20 mg/mL (Roche Bio-chemicals, West Sussex, UK).

2.2   Equipment

No specialized laboratory equipment is required to follow the HmeDIP protocol. We have listed standard laboratory apparatus used as well as the specific models employed in our laboratory, although equivalent devices may be used:

1. Spectrophotometer: NanoDrop™ 8000 (Thermo Scientific, DE, USA).

2. Benchtop hot-block: Thermomixer comfort (Eppendorf, UK).

3. Sonicator: Bioruptor® Standard - chilled (Diagenode®, NJ, USA).

4. Test tube rotator: LD-79 (Labinco BV, Breda, Netherlands).

5. Magnetic rack: DynaMag™-2 (Life Technologies, Paisley, UK).

3   Methods

3.1   DNA Fragmentation by Sonication

1. Dilute 20 µg genomic DNA in 400 µl of TE in a flip cap 1.5 mL Eppendorf tube. Perform this step on ice (*see* **Note 1**).

2. Place samples in a prechilled (4 °C) sonicator and shear DNA for eight cycles of 30 s ON/30 s OFF on "high" (*see* **Note 2**).

3. Determine the DNA concentration of the sonicated samples accurately. Take multiple measurements of each sample where sample material is plentiful (*see* **Note 3**). Run approximately 250 ng of sonicated DNA on a 1.5 % agarose gel for 1.5 h at 100 V (*see* **Note 4**). The size range of the smear should be approximately 200–1000 bp, with a modal size of 500–700 bp (*see* **Note 5**).

3.2   Hydroxy-methylated DNA Immunoprecipitation (hmeDIP)

1. Dilute 4 µg sonicated DNA in 450 µl TE in a 1.5 mL screw-top tube.

2. [Optional] Spike in a 5hmC rich DNA template to act as a positive control for immunoprecipitation of 5hmC-containing DNA (*see* **Note 6**).

3. Denature DNA by incubation at 100 °C for 10 min in a hot-block, followed by snap-chilling samples on wet-ice for 5 min (*see* **Notes 7** and **8**). Collect sample by brief centrifugation in a chilled centrifuge and place on ice.

4. Transfer 45 µl of denatured sample to a fresh 1.5 mL tube. This sample will serve as the "input" control for the IP sample.

5. Add 45 µl 10× IP buffer to remaining sample, followed by 2 µl of α-5hmC antibody (ActiveMotif, CA, USA) (*see* **Note 9**).

6. Incubate samples for 3 h at 4 °C on a rotating wheel at 25 rpm (*see* **Note 10**).

7. Shortly before the end of the incubation period, prepare and wash 40 µl Dynabeads Protein G (30 mg/mL) per sample in a new 1.5 mL flip cap Eppendorf tube (*see* **Note 11**).

8. Wash Dynabeads in 800 mL PBS-BSA for 5 min on a rotating wheel at room temperature. Remove the liquid by placing the tube in a magnetic rack and carefully pipetting off the wash solution.

9. Resuspend the washed beads in 40 µl of 1× IP buffer (4 °C).

10. Once the antibody is complete, add 40 µl of the Dynabead mixture and incubate for 1 h on a rotating wheel at 4 °C (*see* **Note 12**).

11. Collect the beads with the magnetic rack and aspirate the supernatant (*see* **Note 13**).

12. Wash the beads with 1 mL 1× IP buffer (4 °C) for 5 min on a rotating wheel at room temperature. Collect the beads using the magnetic rack and discard the supernatant. Repeat this step three times in total (*see* **Note 14**).

13. To release the DNA from the beads, resuspend the beads in 250 µl digestion buffer, and add 10 µl Proteinase K (20 mg/mL stock). Incubate samples for a minimum of 3 h at 50 °C (or overnight) in a shaking heat block at 800 rpm (*see* **Note 15**).

14. Purify the immunoprecipitated DNA (IP sample) fragments *and* the INPUT sample using a PCR purification column or by phenol–chloroform extraction followed by ethanol precipitation (*see* **Note 16**). Resuspend or elute in 45 µl of TE.

15. Subsequently, 3 µl of the INPUT and IP samples are used as templates in quantitative PCR. qPCR parameters will vary with machine type, assay type, and PCR primer efficiency. Typically, the enrichment values are displayed as IP copy number/INPUT copy number as determined by qPCR. For human brain and liver tissues, *H19* and *Tex19.1* promoter loci can be used as positive endogenous control loci, while the *GAPDH* promoter can be used as a negative endogenous control locus) (*see* **Note 17**).

4   Notes

1. It is important to ensure that the genomic DNA used is free from contaminating agents and does not show signs of degradation. We have optimized this protocol for use with 20 µg DNA, which allows for several HmeDIPs from the same sonicated material. If the DNA is limiting, as little as 2.0 µg can be used, however, sonication conditions will have to be optimized for altered DNA concentrations. Always keep 250 ng of the

sonicated sample to run on an agarose gel to check for fragmentation.

2. It is critical to optimize this step for the machine used and the amount of starting DNA. We typically find that eight cycles, 30 s on/off on a high setting works well on our Diagenode Bioruptor®. Before starting this protocol it is imperative that sonication conditions are established to obtain DNA fragments ranging from 200 to 1000 bp, with the majority fragmented to ~500 bp in size.

3. Although each sample should have a similar DNA concentration, due to the viscosity of genomic DNA the actual amount of DNA added to each sample may vary. It is therefore important to determine sample concentrations after sonication.

4. Gel running conditions may vary depending upon the apparatus used. Optimize gel electrophoresis conditions to obtain good resolution in the range of 100–1500 bp.

5. It is not uncommon for the fragmentation profiles to differ slightly between samples. This is fine so long as the general fragment size range is the same for all samples (i.e., the majority of DNA is between 200 and 1000 bp peaking at 500 bp). It is not advised to perform HmeDIP on samples exhibiting significantly different fragment size ranges. If required, an extra pulse of sonication can be performed on samples requiring further fragmentation. We suggest that samples to be compared by hmeDIP be sonicated simultaneously to reduce inter-sample variation in fragment size.

6. Our knowledge of locus-specific quantities of 5hmC in mammalian genomes is still rather limited, as is our knowledge of how these levels vary between tissues. Thus, in the absence of endogenous positive control regions, the addition of an exogenous 5hmC-DNA positive control is highly recommended. 5hmC control templates are made by amplification of DNA in which canonical dCTP has been replaced by hydroxymethyl dCTP (dhmCTP) in the polymerase chain reaction (PCR). Any short (200–1000 bp), CpG rich DNA template may be used to generate the 5hmC control. Note that all cytosines in the amplified product will be hydroxymethylcytosine, not just those in the context of a CpG. To accurately mimic a hydroxymethylated single-copy locus in the genome, the number of control molecules added should be equal to the number of haploid genomes in the hmeDIP [13]. 5hmC-containing control DNA is also available commercially (New England Biolabs, CA, USA and Zymo Research, CA, USA). We recently reported endogenous regions at the *IGF2/H19* imprinted locus that were relatively enriched for 5hmC in eight normal human tissues and several cell lines [9]. These loci may be used as

endogenous positive control regions. However, as the region is imprinted, 5hmC content may vary with developmental stage. The unmethylated CpG islands of housekeeping genes such as *GAPDH* and *ACTB* may be used as negative control regions.

7. Denaturation of the DNA is not required as the 5hmC antibody employed here also recognizes dsDNA (double stranded DNA); however, its sensitivity is significantly higher for ssDNA (single stranded DNA). Thus, using the same conditions for denaturation for every sample is important as varying amounts of ssDNA to dsDNA between samples may affect antibody binding affinity and consequently enrichment values. Snap-chilling on wet-ice is important, given the large sample volume; thin-walled tubes should be used if possible.

8. It is important at this stage to determine if one requires double or single stranded DNA for downstream applications. Although it is possible to purify double stranded DNA for genome wide sequencing without denaturation, we do not recommend this, as the final yield will be low and thus hard to prepare libraries from. Instead we suggest that any genome wide sequencing adapters are ligated on prior to this stage and denaturation and DIP carried out on these adapter mediated DNA fragments.

9. Although several 5hmC antibodies are currently available, we and others have found the polyclonal 5hmC antibody from ActiveMotif to be the most sensitive and specific of those available [5, 6, 25, 26]. Be aware that the whole serum or purified IgG versions of the antibody have very different titres. We used the IgG purified version in this method. Each batch of antibody should be tested, as different batches of a polyclonal antibody can have very different binding affinities for the epitope.

10. Overnight incubation can be used; however, this may increase nonspecific binding.

11. Using Dynabeads Protein A instead of Dynabeads Protein G (Life Technologies, Paisley, UK) will give similar results.

12. Longer incubations times can result in increased nonspecific binding of DNA to the beads.

13. The supernatant, or "flow-through," contains the DNA not bound by the antibody, and thus depleted for 5hmC. This can be retained to assay regions depleted for 5hmC.

14. The wash steps serve to remove any contaminating DNA not bound to the antibody, and thus reduce the signal-to-noise ratio in the results.

15. The samples are shaken to prevent the beads from sedimenting at the bottom of the tube and consequently reducing the efficiency of the proteinase reaction. It is recommended to

perform this step overnight; however, a 3 h incubation is also sufficient.

16. We use the QIAquick PCR kit (QIAgen, Crawley, UK) to purify the INPUT sample and IP sample DNA, eluting in 47 μl of TE, to yield a final volume of 45 μl. We found this approach gave best reproducibility between experiments.

17. Unlike global 5mC levels, which are broadly similar between mammalian tissues, we and others have shown that global 5hmC levels vary markedly between tissue types [9, 27]. For example, normal human breast has a lower global 5hmC content than normal human brain and consequently shows lower enrichment values at all endogenous loci tested. Thus, inter-tissue differences in global 5hmC content should be considered when designing hmeDIP experiments.

As with 5mC antibodies, 5hmC antibodies exhibit slight sequence-biases in their binding affinities [24]. Given the lack of high quality genome-wide, quantitative data for 5hmC, the extent of such effects, if any, is difficult to determine at present. A meta-analysis of genome-wide 5hmC profiles determined by hmeDIP and other 5hmC profiling techniques suggested that the antibody used here may bind unmethylated CA- and CT-, but this cross-reactivity has yet to be confirmed [24, 28].

Acknowledgements

We thank Dr. Jamie Hackett for his role in initially developing the hmeDIP protocol presented here. Research in RRMs lab is supported by the Medical Research Council, the BBSRC and IMI-MARCAR: the Innovative Medicine Initiative Joint Undertaking (IMI JU) under grant agreement number 115001 (MARCAR project. URL: http://www.imi-marcar.eu/).

References

1. Kriaucionis S, Heintz N (2009) The nuclear DNA base 5-hydroxymethylcytosine is present in Purkinje neurons and the brain. Science 324:929–930

2. Shen L, Zhang Y (2013) 5-hydroxymethylcytosine: generation, fate, and genomic distribution. Curr Opin Cell Biol 25 (3):289–296

3. Song CX, Yi C, He C (2012) Mapping recently identified nucleotide variants in the genome and transcriptome. Nat Biotechnol 30:1107–1116

4. Tahiliani M, Koh KP, Shen Y, Pastor WA, Bandukwala H, Brudno Y, Agarwal S, Iyer LM, Liu DR, Aravind L et al (2009) Conversion of 5-methylcytosine to 5-hydroxymethylcytosine in mammalian DNA by MLL partner TET1. Science 324:930–935

5. Thomson JP, Hunter JM, Lempiainen H, Muller A, Terranova R, Moggs JG, Meehan RR (2013) Dynamic changes in 5-hydroxymethylation signatures underpin early and late events in drug exposed liver. Nucleic Acids Res 41:5639–5654

6. Thomson JP, Lempiainen H, Hackett JA, Nestor CE, Muller A, Bolognani F, Oakeley EJ, Schubeler D, Terranova R, Reinhardt D et al (2012) Non-genotoxic carcinogen exposure

induces defined changes in the 5-hydroxymethylome. Genome Biol 13:R93

7. Robinson MD, Stirzaker C, Statham AL, Coolen MW, Song JZ, Nair SS, Strbenac D, Speed TP, Clark SJ (2010) Evaluation of affinity-based genome-wide DNA methylation data: effects of CpG density, amplification bias, and copy number variation. Genome Res 20:1719–1729

8. Globisch D, Munzel M, Muller M, Michalakis S, Wagner M, Koch S, Bruckl T, Biel M, Carell T (2010) Tissue distribution of 5-hydroxymethylcytosine and search for active demethylation intermediates. PLoS One 5:e15367

9. Nestor CE, Ottaviano R, Reddington J, Sproul D, Reinhardt D, Dunican D, Katz E, Dixon JM, Harrison DJ, Meehan RR (2012) Tissue type is a major modifier of the 5-hydroxymethylcytosine content of human genes. Genome Res 22:467–477

10. Laird A, Thomson JP, Harrison DJ, Meehan RR (2013) 5-hydroxymethylcytosine profiling as an indicator of cellular state. Epigenomics 5:655–669

11. Thomson JP, Moggs JG, Wolf CR, Meehan RR (2013) Epigenetic profiles as defined signatures of xenobiotic exposure. Mutat Res Genet Toxicol Environ Mutagen 764–765:3–9

12. Ficz G, Gribben JG (2014) Loss of 5-hydroxymethylcytosine in cancer: cause or consequence? Genomics 104(5):352–357

13. Nestor C, Ruzov A, Meehan R, Dunican D (2010) Enzymatic approaches and bisulfite sequencing cannot distinguish between 5-methylcytosine and 5-hydroxymethylcytosine in DNA. Biotechniques 48:317–319

14. Huang Y, Pastor WA, Zepeda-Martinez JA, Rao A (2012) The anti-CMS technique for genome-wide mapping of 5-hydroxymethylcytosine. Nat Protoc 7:1897–1908

15. Cui L, Chung TH, Tan D, Sun X, Jia XY (2014) JBP1-seq: a fast and efficient method for genome-wide profiling of 5hmC. Genomics 104:368–375

16. Robertson AB, Dahl JA, Ougland R, Klungland A (2012) Pull-down of 5-hydroxymethylcytosine DNA using JBP1-coated magnetic beads. Nat Protoc 7:340–350

17. Song CX, Szulwach KE, Fu Y, Dai Q, Yi C, Li X, Li Y, Chen CH, Zhang W, Jian X et al (2011) Selective chemical labeling reveals the genome-wide distribution of 5-hydroxymethylcytosine. Nat Biotechnol 29:68–72

18. Serandour AA, Avner S, Oger F, Bizot M, Percevault F, Lucchetti-Miganeh C, Palierne G, Gheeraert C, Barloy-Hubler F, Peron CL et al (2012) Dynamic hydroxymethylation of deoxyribonucleic acid marks differentiation-associated enhancers. Nucleic Acids Res 40:8255–8265

19. Szulwach KE, Li X, Li Y, Song CX, Wu H, Dai Q, Irier H, Upadhyay AK, Gearing M, Levey AI et al (2011) 5-hmC-mediated epigenetic dynamics during postnatal neurodevelopment and aging. Nat Neurosci 14:1607–1616

20. Wang T, Wu H, Li Y, Szulwach KE, Lin L, Li X, Chen IP, Goldlust IS, Chamberlain SJ, Dodd A et al (2013) Subtelomeric hotspots of aberrant 5-hydroxymethylcytosine-mediated epigenetic modifications during reprogramming to pluripotency. Nat Cell Biol 15:700–711

21. Booth MJ, Branco MR, Ficz G, Oxley D, Krueger F, Reik W, Balasubramanian S (2012) Quantitative sequencing of 5-methylcytosine and 5-hydroxymethylcytosine at single-base resolution. Science 336:934–937

22. Yu M, Hon GC, Szulwach KE, Song CX, Zhang L, Kim A, Li X, Dai Q, Shen Y, Park B et al (2012) Base-resolution analysis of 5-hydroxymethylcytosine in the mammalian genome. Cell 149:1368–1380

23. Booth MJ, Ost TW, Beraldi D, Bell NM, Branco MR, Reik W, Balasubramanian S (2013) Oxidative bisulfite sequencing of 5-methylcytosine and 5-hydroxymethylcytosine. Nat Protoc 8:1841–1851

24. Thomson JP, Hunter JM, Nestor CE, Dunican DS, Terranova R, Moggs JG, Meehan RR (2013) Comparative analysis of affinity-based 5-hydroxymethylation enrichment techniques. Nucleic Acids Res 41:e206

25. Ficz G, Branco MR, Seisenberger S, Santos F, Krueger F, Hore TA, Marques CJ, Andrews S, Reik W (2011) Dynamic regulation of 5-hydroxymethylcytosine in mouse ES cells and during differentiation. Nature 473:398–402

26. Wu H, D'Alessio AC, Ito S, Wang Z, Cui K, Zhao K, Sun YE, Zhang Y (2011) Genome-wide analysis of 5-hydroxymethylcytosine distribution reveals its dual function in transcriptional regulation in mouse embryonic stem cells. Genes Dev 25:679–684

27. Szwagierczak A, Bultmann S, Schmidt CS, Spada F, Leonhardt H (2010) Sensitive enzymatic quantification of 5-hydroxymethylcytosine in genomic DNA. Nucleic Acids Res 38:e181

28. Matarese F, Carrillo-de Santa Pau E, Stunnenberg HG (2011) 5-hydroxymethylcytosine: a new kid on the epigenetic block? Mol Syst Biol 7:562

Methods in Molecular Biology (2017) 1589: 99–106
DOI 10.1007/7651_2015_262
© Springer Science+Business Media New York 2015
Published online: 01 July 2016

Adjusting for Cell Type Composition in DNA Methylation Data Using a Regression-Based Approach

Meaghan J. Jones, Sumaiya A. Islam, Rachel D. Edgar, and Michael S. Kobor

Abstract

Analysis of DNA methylation in a population context has the potential to uncover novel gene and environment interactions as well as markers of health and disease. In order to find such associations it is important to control for factors which may mask or alter DNA methylation signatures. Since tissue of origin and coinciding cell type composition are major contributors to DNA methylation patterns, and can easily confound important findings, it is vital to adjust DNA methylation data for such differences across individuals. Here we describe the use of a regression method to adjust for cell type composition in DNA methylation data. We specifically discuss what information is required to adjust for cell type composition and then provide detailed instructions on how to perform cell type adjustment on high dimensional DNA methylation data. This method has been applied mainly to Illumina 450K data, but can also be adapted to pyrosequencing or genome-wide bisulfite sequencing data.

Keywords: DNA methylation, Illumina Infinium HumanMethylation450 BeadChip, Cell type, Statistical adjustment, R statistical software

1 Introduction

The number of DNA methylation studies in human populations has been steadily and rapidly rising and this trend will likely continue. With this increase, there is growing appreciation for stringency in analysis and a more complete understanding of important factors to consider when analyzing DNA methylation data. One factor which is now understood to be important is adjusting for interindividual differences in cell type composition of the tissue being interrogated [1–5].

Since, within a tissue, cell type is the single most important known factor in determining DNA methylation profiles, it then follows that differences in interindividual composition of cell types might significantly confound results from DNA methylation analyses [1–3, 5]. For example, if the phenotype of interest is associated with a change in cell composition in the tissue being examined, not adjusting for these differences could result in identification of cell type-specific regions as being associated with the phenotype. This issue has been specifically described in studies of rheumatoid arthritis, age, and current socioeconomic status, where in all three cases, differences in cell type composition of white blood cells between individuals were confounded with the phenotype of interest [2–4]. This would have led to many potential false positives had the researchers not accounted for these differences. Even if the phenotype of interest is not confounded by cell type differences, the large amount of variability due to these differences can alter or mask true associations; therefore adjustment of DNA methylation data for interindividual differences in cell type composition should still be performed. It is worth noting that such adjustments should be performed within a single tissue (i.e., brain samples) and not across different tissue types (i.e., blood versus brain samples).

Many studies have highlighted the need for cell type composition adjustment in tissues composed of multiple cell types [2–4, 6, 7]. However, not all tissues have received the same scrutiny and not all available methods are appropriate for every tissue. For example, the most commonly used surrogate tissues are buccal epithelial cells (BEC) and blood. Both of these tissues are composed of multiple cell types; blood contains a multitude of white blood cells, while BECs can have some contaminating level of blood or other tissues [7]. However, while most recent DNA methylation studies using blood include adjustment for cell type composition differences, adjustment of BECs has been attempted in only a few cases [7, 8]. It is also important to acknowledge that in a mixed cell population, a change in DNA methylation that is restricted to an underrepresented cell subtype may not be detected, regardless of adjustment. These changes may be highly interesting, but can only be detected if the tissue is fractionated to separate the cell types.

Here, we describe a regression method to adjust for cell type composition in DNA methylation data. This method is appropriate for use in cases where cell type counts are available, often through direct measurement. In the absence of direct cell counts, various cell type composition prediction methods have been established [6, 9, 10]. Current prediction methods are focused on blood and brain, but in the future other tissues may receive the same scrutiny. Although the computational details for each of these prediction algorithms are beyond the scope of our discussion, it is worth noting that these methods primarily utilize differential DNA methylation signatures of each constituent cell type as references to generate projections of cell type proportions in a given tissue. In this chapter, we will first outline how to decide whether this method is applicable to the specific study and then describe the procedure to follow to adjust the data for differences in cell type between individuals. This regression method is a robust approach to adjust for such differences in cell type composition and accordingly represents an appreciable contribution to the increasing rigor of DNA methylation analyses.

2   Materials

Several pieces of information are required to control for cellular composition of a tissue sample using the regression method:

2.1   Cell Counts

Cell counts can come from a variety of sources, which may vary depending on the tissue (*see* **Note 1**). For histological samples, approximate counts from microscopy may be appropriate. For blood, cell counts are often generated by lab-derived Complete Blood Count (CBC, *see* **Note 2**) with differential reports or by fluorescence-activated cell sorting (FACS) analysis (*see* **Note 3**).

If a cell count from the tissue is unavailable, published methods exist for predicting the underlying cellular composition based on the DNA methylation profile of the tissue for blood and brain [6, 9–11]. These methods have been used extensively and have proven to be highly reliable in many cases (*see* **Note 4**). In the script below, cell counts are contained in an object called "diff", which is a matrix of cell counts with samples as rows, and cell types as columns (*see* **Note 1**).

2.2   DNA Methylation Profiles

Described here is the method commonly used for adjustment of DNA methylation data generated by the Illumina 450K array (*see* **Note 5**). For 450K analysis, we recommend that cellular composition adjustment be done after initial preprocessing and quality control checks including probe filtering, normalization, and batch correction according to the pipeline of choice. The input into the script below is an object called "betas" (*see* **Note 6**), which is a matrix of beta values with CpG probes as rows and samples as columns in the same order as the rows in the diff matrix (*see* **Note 7**).

2.3   Statistical Software

R statistical software with R-specific script is commonly used for this method (*see* **Note 8**) [12].

3   Methods

First, a decision must be made regarding whether the regression method can be applied to the specific project in question, or whether reference-free methods must be used (*see* **Note 9**). A flow chart is laid out in Fig. 1 illustrating the best choices for particular projects. Importantly, this should only be used if there is reason to expect that the tissue being assessed contains a mixture of cell types which might differ across individuals.

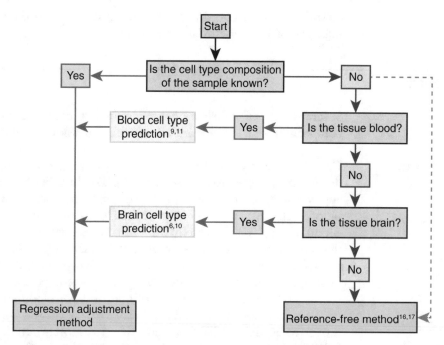

Fig. 1 Flow chart describing decision tree to determine whether cell type adjustment using the regression/residual method is appropriate, or whether a reference-free method should be used (methods in *purple*). The regression method outlined in this chapter can be used in any case where the cellular composition of the sample is known or can be predicted (with blood or brain prediction algorithms, shown in *yellow*)

Once the appropriate information has been gathered, as outlined in Section 2, you can proceed to adjust DNA methylation data for cell composition differences using the regression method. The process to adjust the data is as follows, with the appropriate R code and annotation.

1.
```
beta.lm<-apply(betas, 1, function(x){diff[colnames
(betas),]->blood

lm(x~CD8T+CD4T+NK+Bcell+Mono+Gran,data=blood)})
```

First, for each probe in the beta matrix, fit a linear model on the DNA methylation measures using cell type proportions as additive variables (here illustrated using blood cell types, *see* **Notes 2, 10,** and **11**). This estimates the degree of DNA methylation variability that is predicted by the underlying cell type composition for each probe.

2.
```
residuals<-t(sapply(beta.lm,function(x)residuals
(summary(x))))

colnames(residuals)<-colnames(betas)
```

Next, extract a matrix of residuals from the resulting linear models. For each probe, the residuals are calculated as the difference between the observed methylation values and predicted methylation values from the fitted linear model. These residuals represent the remaining DNA methylation

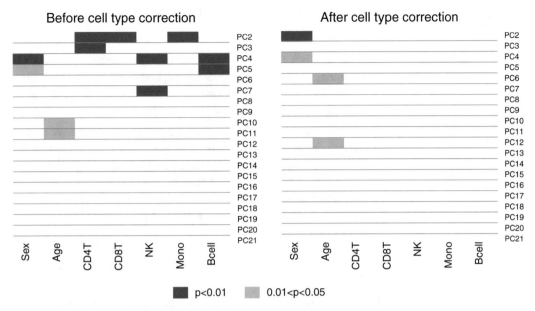

Fig. 2 Illustration of ideal results after using PCA to assess the effect of adjusting DNA methylation data for cell type composition. Heatmap indicates *p* values of correlations between the top 20 Principal Components (PCs) and variables. Prior to cell type adjustment (*left*), many of the top PCs are associated with cell types, some of which are confounded with sex and age (serving as example test variables). After cell type adjustment (*right*) the associations with cell type are no longer observed, but the signal from the two test variables is still clear

variability that are unexplained by cell type composition and may accordingly be explained by other phenotypic factors of interest. Since a linear model is fit to each probe individually, sites with methylation levels that are less affected by cell type composition will accordingly be modified to a lesser extent than a probe that is highly associated with cell type composition.

3. `adj.betas<-residuals+matrix(apply(betas, 1, mean), nrow=nrow(residuals), ncol=ncol(residuals))`

Next, add the residuals of each regression model to the mean methylation value of each probe (mean across all samples) to obtain the "adjusted" methylation data.

4. `adj.m<-beta2m(adj.betas)`

Finally, and optionally, perform a logit transformation to convert the beta values back to *M* values for downstream statistical analysis using the beta2m function in the lumi R package (*see* **Note 12**) [13].

5. (Optional) Perform Principal Component Analysis (PCA) on the original beta value matrix and the adjusted beta values to determine whether any variation associated with cell type has been removed from the data (*see* **Note 13**). An example of how this should appear is shown in Fig. 2.

4 Notes

1. Cell counts can be represented as either proportions (in percent) or absolute cell counts, but these should be treated differently when fitting the linear models in **Step 1** of the regression method, as described in **Note 10**.

2. Whole blood samples are often fractionated to remove granulocytes, resulting in an enriched population of mononuclear cells, prior to DNA methylation analysis. It should be noted that a lab-generated CBC differential report from whole blood may not accurately reflect the cellular composition of mononuclear cells isolated from the same sample. Thus, for mononuclear cells, if post-mononuclear cell enrichment counts are not available, it is generally recommended that blood cell type prediction methods be used to generate accurate cell counts [9, 11, 14].

3. FACS-derived counts are often highly accurate representations of actual cellular composition of a sample; however particular care must be taken with the staining and isolation of cells to ensure that artifacts are not introduced. For example, specifically increased mortality of a single cell type in the preparation could skew the results and underestimate the true proportions of those cells.

4. The commonly used deconvolution methods for DNA methylation are available for brain and blood, the former found in the CETS R package and the latter in the minfi R package [6, 9, 14]. Both these packages output a matrix of cell counts for each sample. A new method for deconvolution for brain is also available [10]. While highly reliable for samples from adults, it is possible that the blood deconvolution in particular is less accurate for pediatric samples. There is also a possibility that ethnicity, environment, or health status may affect the accuracy of these predictions, if these factors greatly affect reference methylation profiles at sites used for the prediction. Thus, care should be taken when applying these methods to samples to ensure that confounding factors are not affecting the quality of cell type prediction. If cell counts are available for a subset of samples, or for similar samples, cross-validating the prediction with the known cell composition is an important check.

5. In addition to Illumina 450K array data, this same procedure should be applicable to pyrosequencing, Reduced Representation Bisulfite Sequencing (RRBS) or Whole Genome Bisulfite Sequencing (WGBS) data.

6. Beta values are between 0 and 1, where 0 represents 0 % DNA methylation and 1 represents 100 % methylation. Due to heteroscedasticity of beta values, M values are often used for

statistical analysis [15]. For cell type adjustment, beta values are the appropriate measure, but they should be converted back to M values prior to downstream analysis.

7. Missing values (NAs) in the beta value matrix must be imputed prior to fitting the linear models. Any missing values can be replaced by the probe median value before **Step 1** and the NAs should be replaced after **Step 3**.

8. Although we have described the method using R statistical software and scripts, the regression method should be adaptable to any software package.

9. If no cell count is available or predictable for the tissue in question (i.e., tissue is not blood or brain) and there is reasonable expectation that cell type composition would differ between individuals, reference-free methods or surrogate variable methods may be the best choice [16–18]. However, these methods have some limitations. They have been specifically designed for array analysis and may not be transferable to RRBS or WGBS data. These reference-free methods in particular are also designed as full analysis packages, with little control or oversight into the intervening steps.

10. If absolute cell counts are used in the regression method, all counted cell types should be included in the model. However, if percent proportions are used, where all the cell types counted add to 100 %, one of the cell type columns should be removed to serve as the intercept and avoid over-fitting. Note that the lm function in R automatically removes one of these columns by default if the values are in percent (*see* **Step 1** in Section 3).

11. It is important to note that the regression method adjusts the data independently of other covariates, resulting in a matrix of beta or M values in which the effects of cell composition have been removed. This is slightly different from another common method, which is to add the cell type variables as covariates in the linear modes used in the analysis itself [4]. We feel that the regression method is superior in most cases because downstream analyses are not required to include cell type variables each time. This is helpful for analyses using methods where incorporation of extra variables is difficult, such as hierarchical clustering.

12. After cell type adjustment, some beta values may have been scaled to numbers higher than 1 or lower than 0. It is important to change these numbers before converting to M values, as they will result in values of infinity or $-$infinity when converted. Our procedure is to replace any numbers higher than 1 with the highest value that is less than one, and similarly to replace any values lower than 0 with the lowest non-negative number.

13. In the specific case where cell type composition is confounded with a variable of interest, it should be apparent in the PCA analysis. This represents a potentially highly interesting aspect of the phenotype, but does complicate DNA methylation studies. Adjusting the data for cell type composition is extremely important in a case such as this, but it is important to be aware that the adjustment may remove some of the DNA methylation signal associated with the phenotype. In order to find pure signals associated with the phenotype, purification of a single cell type may be required.

References

1. Reinius LE, Acevedo N, Joerink M et al (2012) Differential DNA methylation in purified human blood cells: implications for cell lineage and studies on disease susceptibility. PLoS One 7:e41361

2. Jaffe AE, Irizarry RA (2014) Accounting for cellular heterogeneity is critical in epigenome wide association studies. Genome Biol 15:R31

3. Lam LL, Emberly E, Fraser HB et al (2012) Factors underlying variable DNA methylation in a human community cohort. Proc Natl Acad Sci U S A 109(Suppl 2):17253–17260

4. Liu Y, Aryee MJ, Padyukov L et al (2013) Epigenome-wide association data implicate DNA methylation as an intermediary of genetic risk in rheumatoid arthritis. Nat Biotechnol 31:142–147

5. Lowe R, Rakyan VK (2014) Correcting for cell-type composition bias in epigenome-wide association studies. Genome Med 6:23

6. Guintivano J, Aryee MJ, Kaminsky ZA (2013) A cell epigenotype specific model for the correction of brain cellular heterogeneity bias and its application to age, brain region and major depression. Epigenetics 8:290–302

7. Jones MJ, Farré P, McEwen LM et al (2013) Distinct DNA methylation patterns of cognitive impairment and trisomy 21 in down syndrome. BMC Med Genomics 6:58

8. Smith AK, Kilaru V, Klengel T et al (2014) DNA extracted from saliva for methylation studies of psychiatric traits: evidence tissue specificity and relatedness to brain. Am J Med Genet 168:36–44

9. Houseman EA, Accomando WP, Koestler DC et al (2012) DNA methylation arrays as surrogate measures of cell mixture distribution. BMC Bioinform 13:86

10. Montaño CM, Irizarry RA, Kaufmann WE et al (2013) Measuring cell-type specific differential methylation in human brain tissue. Genome Biol 14:R94

11. Koestler DC, Christensen B, Karagas MR et al (2013) Blood-based profiles of DNA methylation predict the underlying distribution of cell types: a validation analysis. Epigenetics 8:816–826

12. D.C.T. R (2008) R: a language and environment for statistical computing. R Foundation for Statistical Computing, Vienna

13. Du P, Kibbe WA, Lin SM (2008) lumi: a pipeline for processing Illumina microarray. Bioinformatics 24:1547–1548

14. Aryee MJ, Jaffe AE, Corrada-Bravo H et al (2014) Minfi: a flexible and comprehensive Bioconductor package for the analysis of Infinium DNA methylation microarrays. Bioinformatics 30:1363–1369

15. Du P, Zhang X, Huang C-C et al (2010) Comparison of Beta-value and M-value methods for quantifying methylation levels by microarray analysis. BMC Bioinform 11:587

16. Zou J, Lippert C, Heckerman D et al (2014) Epigenome-wide association studies without the need for cell-type composition. Nat Methods 11:309–311

17. Houseman EA, Molitor J, Marsit CJ (2014) Reference-free cell mixture adjustments in analysis of DNA methylation data. Bioinformatics 30:1431–1439

18. Leek JT, Johnson WE, Parker HS et al (2012) The sva package for removing batch effects and other unwanted variation in high-throughput experiments. Bioinformatics 28:882–883

Methods in Molecular Biology (2017) 1589: 107–114
DOI 10.1007/7651_2015_266
© Springer Science+Business Media New York 2015
Published online: 06 August 2016

Correcting for Sample Heterogeneity in Methylome-Wide Association Studies

James Y. Zou

Abstract

Epigenome-wide association studies (EWAS) face many of the same challenges as genome-wide association studies (GWAS), but have an added challenge in that the epigenome can vary dramatically across cell types. When cell-type composition differs between cases and controls, this leads to spurious associations that may obscure true associations. We have developed a computational method, FaST-LMM-EWASher, which automatically corrects for cell-type composition without needing explicit knowledge of it. In this chapter, we provide a tutorial on using FaST-LMM-EWASher for DNA methylation data and discuss data analysis strategies.

Keywords: DNA methylation, Epigenome-wide association study, Computational method, Sample heterogeneity

1 Introduction

With the era of next-generation sequencing comes high-throughput measurement not only of the genome but also of the epigenome, yielding complementary information that is critical to the understanding of disease mechanisms. Epigenetics informs us about the structure and accessibility of DNA, which in turn yields information about regulation and transcription—key drivers of disease. Thus, epigenetics is a crucial mediating link between genetics and function. In many diseases, it is now appreciated that both epigenetic changes and genetic factors influence disease risk [1–4].

Currently, the measurement and analysis of epigenetic data through epigenome-wide association studies (EWAS) is a subject of considerable interest as such analyses yield insights into the role of epigenetic regulation in disease [5]. The goal of EWAS, analogous to GWAS, is to identify changes in the epigenome at particular loci that are correlated with some phenotype of interest, by scanning along the entire epigenome. While such analysis alone cannot establish causality, epigenetic association studies shed light on disease pathways and drivers and also identify candidate biomarkers for diagnostics [5].

The shared challenges in EWAS and GWAS include confounding by batch effects, population structure and family relatedness, adjusted for multiple hypothesis testing, and the need to group together weak effects to find underpowered associations [6, 7]. Importantly, EWAS faces the additional, significant challenge in that the epigenome can be highly variable across different cell types [8], and case and control samples in a study may well differ in their cell-type compositions. Such heterogeneity can give rise to spurious associations; see for example a study of methylation in rheumatoid arthritis (Fig. 1) (RA) [9].

One approach to tackle this problem is to measure in each sample the composition of the relevant cell types. For special cases such as whole blood, the cell-type composition of each sample can also be estimated statistically [10]. This composition information

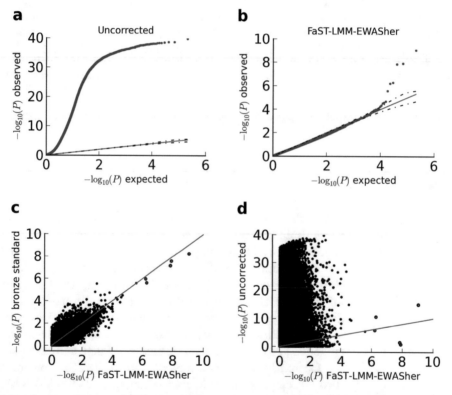

Fig. 1 Illustration of EWASher on the rheumatoid arthritis data. In preprocessing, data were corrected for gender, batch, and smoking status. (**a**) Quantile-quantile (qq) plot of the $-\log_{10} P$ values for association without additional corrections. It shows severely inflated test statistics leading to many false positives. *Black dashed lines* show the 95 % confidence intervals. Large deviations from the diagonal are indicative of inflation. (**b**) qq plot resulting from use of EWASher, which did not use knowledge of cell-type composition. (**c**) Paired plot of the $-\log_{10} P$ values from EWASher and the bronze standard obtained from explicitly using cell-type composition. The two approaches found the exact same five significant loci (with the same rankings). (**d**) Paired plot of the values from (**a**) and (**b**), showing that the correction dramatically altered the rank order of the hypotheses, and that in the uncorrected method, the significant loci were swamped by spurious associations

can then be included as a covariate in the association analysis as demonstrated in the RA study [9]. However, it is difficult to accurately measure or estimate the cell-type composition of each sample, particularly for solid tissues in which pure populations of cells are problematic to obtain.

We have a method—FaST-LMM-EWASher (or EWASher for short)—to automatically adjust for cell-type heterogeneity in DNA methylation data without requiring explicit information about cell-type compositions [11]. This allows us to perform methylation association studies and remove spurious associations. EWASher is a hybrid approach of (1) a feature-selected LMM [12–15] and (2) a principal components (PC) based approach [16, 17]. As we have demonstrated on real and synthetic data, this method successfully corrects for confounding by cell-type composition, without any dependence on purified reference cell types, making it "reference-free." Furthermore, the method is computationally efficient, scaling up to the large datasets produced with current technologies.

EWAS confounding by cell-type composition arises because the cell-type composition is correlated with the phenotype, and also with many methylation loci. As a result, loci that are indicative of cell type will appear to be associated with the phenotype even though they are only correlated by way of cell-type composition. To alleviate this problem, we use the dataset itself to implicitly estimate and correct for this confounding. We use the genome-wide methylation data to construct a single similarity score between every two individuals. Jointly, these similarity scores are reflective of the relative cell-type composition among individuals—two individuals with similar sample cell-type compositions will have a high similarity score, while those with different composition will have a low score. Together, these scores form a similarity matrix, which is then used within the linear mixed model (LMM) to remove associations due to variations in cell-type compositions.

2   Materials

The EWASher software for Windows or Linux can be downloaded at http://research.microsoft.com/en-us/um/redmond/projects/mscompbio/fastlmm/.

Please read the README.txt file and run to the example dataset in the demo folder to ensure that EWASher is working properly on your computer.

The starting point of the analysis is DNA methylation data measured in the same set of loci across samples. Illumina Infinium 27k or 450k DNA methylation chips are popular data platforms. EWASher automatically imputes missing values.

Each sample should be associated with a measured phenotype. The phenotype could be continuous or binary. For example, in case/control study designs—a sample is assigned a phenotype value of 0 if it is a control and 1 if it is a case. The phenotype could also be a real number measuring a quantitative trait. Relevant covariates such as age, gender, and batch of the samples, can be included in the association.

For preprocessing the DNA methylation data, we recommend the R package minfi, which can be downloaded from Bioconductor at: http://www.bioconductor.org/packages/release/bioc/html/minfi.html.

3   Methods

3.1   Preprocessing

The first step is to perform standard QC of the DNA methylation data. This removes bad probes and bad samples and converts the raw data into a β value for each entry. Minfi is an R package that performs this preprocessing, and there are several other programs for doing this.

3.2   Prepare Input

To prepare the input data for EWASher, first prepare separate text files for methylation values, phenotypes, other covariates, and a map file for the locations of the probes. The methylation values and phenotypes are required to run EWASher, while the covariates and the map file are optional. An example set of inputs is included in the demo folder as a part of the download. We describe each of these files in detail.

Table of methylation values. The main input data is a tab-delimited table of methylation values. In 27k and 450k arrays, this corresponds to the beta values of probes. Each column corresponds to a sample and each row corresponds to a probe. The first row is a header: "ID", sampleID1, sampleID2, etc. Each subsequent row has the form: probeID, value1, value2, ...

Phenotype file. Each row has the form: sampleID sampleStatus. For case/control studies, the convention is to set the sample status to 1 if the sample is a case and to 0 otherwise. The sampleID should match the sample IDs in the methylation table. This file is tab delimited.

Covariates [optional]. The user may optionally specify a set of covariates to include in the model (e.g., age, gender). Each row corresponds to a sample. The order of the samples must be the same as in the methylation table header. The first column is always set to "1", the second column is the sample ID, and each subsequent column corresponds to a covariate. Do not add column header. This file is tab delimited.

The map file. EWASher uses the chromosome and genetic distance of every marker. By default, it assumes that the data comes from either the 450k or 27k Illumina Infinium methylation chip, in which case this parameter can be left blank. If the default is not applicable, it is necessary to provide a map file, which contains the chromosome number, name, and genetic distance of each marker, one per row, with no header. The probe locations are used to remove proximal contamination due to correlations of nearby probes. This is a significant problem for GWAS due to linkage disequilibrium and is less of a problem here since the correlations are much smaller.

3.3 Running Ewasher

Place all the input files in one folder. From this folder you can run EWASher by using the command:

```
\PATH\fastlmm-ewasher.py input_data.txt input_phenotype.
txt -covar covariates.txt -map testmarkers.map
```

PATH is the path where the EWASher src folder is saved on your computer, and input_data.txt, input_phenotype.txt, covariates.txt, and testmarkers.map are the names of the four input files. The covariates and map files are optional. If there are no covariates and the standard 450k or 27k arrays have been used simply run:

```
\PATH\fastlmm-ewasher.py input_data.txt input_phenotype.
txt
```

3.4 Outputs of EWASher

EWASher creates two output folders, results/ and tmp/.
   The folder results/ contains the following files:

- *out_ewasher.txt*: The association P values and statistics for each loci as computed by FaST-LMM-EWASher. FaST-LMM-EWASher filters out loci that are constitutively on or off, and the association statistics are computed for the remaining loci.

- *out_linreg.txt*: The P values and statistics from a linear regression with the covariates specified by user.

- *qq_ewasher.png*: This is the qq plot of the FaST-LMM-EWASher P values. Quantile-quantile (qq) plots of the $-\log_{10}P$ quantiles are used to assess inflation of the test statistic experiments, as is common in the GWAS community. In these plots, the quantiles of the theoretical null distribution are plotted against the observed quantiles. Under the assumption that no methylation loci in the observed data are differentially expressed, the resulting plot should follow the diagonal (red line) and lie within the 95 % confidence error bars (black dotted lines). Because we expect some, but not too many, methylation sites to be differentially expressed, we expect to see only small deviations from this, and interpret greater deviations as inflation of the test statistic, potentially leading to more false positive signals [6].

- *qq_linreg.png*: This is the qq plot of the linear regression P values, i.e., the association analysis not correcting for cell-type composition.

- *similarity.txt*: This is the methylome similarity matrix computed and used by EWASher.
- *summary.txt*: A summary file that states how many loci were analyzed and how many principle components were used by EWASher.
- *ASout.snps.txt*: The list of all the markers used to construct the similarity matrix.

The tmp directory contains intermediary files created during the execution of EWASher. Some of these files can be useful for troubleshooting. *See* Section 4 for additional suggestions for common troubleshooting and for future extensions of EWASher. If the linear mixed model alone cannot correct for inflated test statistics, EWASher iteratively adds principle components (PC) until the test statistics are calibrated. If k PCs are selected, then the tmp folder also contains *out_lmm_0.txt*, *out_lmm_1.txt*, ... *out_lmm_k.txt*. Each one shows the results from running EWASher with intermediate number of principle components.

3.5 Interpreting the EWASher Output

The markers are outputted to out_ewasher.txt and are listed in order of *p* value significance. The column "Pvalue" gives the uncorrected *p* value from likelihood ratio test. The next column ("Qvalue") gives the false discovery *Q* values. To get the Bonferroni corrected *p* value, the raw *p* value are multiplied by the number of markers tested.

Investigators can look at the top markers in the out_linreg.txt file to see whether associations remain significant after correcting for cell-type composition. If they are not, this indicates that these are potentially markers that tag specific cell types.

3.6 Downstream Analysis and Functional Enrichments

Gene Ontology analysis. Once a list of significant loci is generated (it is also possible to take the top 100 or 200 loci, even if some of these are below the Bonferroni threshold due to lack of power), potential biological functions associated with these loci may be investigated, for example by assigning the CpG to the nearest gene. Most association CpGs tend to be in the promoter or intron of genes, and in this case it is clear which gene to assign. For intergenic loci, the simplest approach is to assign it to the nearest gene and run standard Gene Ontology analysis on the assigned genes to see what functions are enriched.

GWAS hits overlap/enrichment. If the phenotype of interest has GWAS hits, it is possible to determine if any of the GWAS hits are near the top associated CpGs. In addition, it is also possible to look at known genes and biomarkers to assess if any of these are near the associated CpGs. Significance of this overlap can be assessed by permutation testing.

Visualizing the results. It is useful to make a Manhattan plot of association p values. This is commonly used in GWAS analysis and allows visualization of loci in the same genes or regions that also show correlation with phenotype, but might be below the Bonferroni cutoff. Lastly it is useful to take each of the top CpGs and look at the box plots its β values in cases and controls.

4   Notes

Troubleshooting. EWASher runs on Windows and Linux. It uses the standard Python packages: numpy, scipy, scikit-learn, and pylab.

Extensions. Most of the EWAS studies have focused on DNA methylation because it is a stable mark and there are efficient technology for assessing its values across many loci. With sequencing, it is also possible to study other epigenomic marks such as DNA hypersensitivity and chromatin modifications in appropriate samples across populations. These studies will face similar problems in having to correct for cell-type heterogeneity in these samples, and extensions of EWASher are being developed to work for those settings.

Acknowledgements

FaST-LMM-EWASher was developed in collaboration with Jennifer Listgarten, Martin Aryee, and the Microsoft Research Los Angeles group. We would also like to thank Yvonne Yamanaka for helpful feedback.

References

1. Jones P (2012) Functions of DNA methylation: islands, start sites, gene bodies and beyond. Nat Rev Genet 13:484–492

2. Portela A, Esteller M (2010) Epigenetic modifications and human disease. Nat Biotechnol 28:1057–1068

3. Kulis M, Esteller M (2010) DNA methylation and cancer. Adv Genet 70:27–56

4. Lechner M, Boshoff C, Beck S (2010) Cancer epigenome. Adv Genet 70:247–276

5. Rakyan VK, Down TA, Balding DJ, Beck S (2011) Epigenome-wide association studies for common human diseases. Nat Rev Genet 12:529–541

6. Balding DJ (2006) A tutorial on statistical methods for population association studies. Nat Rev Genet 7:781–791

7. Listgarten J et al (2013) A powerful and efficient set test for genetic markers that handles confounders. Bioinformatics 29:1526–1533

8. Zhu J et al (2013) Genome-wide chromatin state transitions elicited by developmental and environmental cues. Cell 152:642–654

9. Liu Y et al (2013) Epigenome-wide association data implicate DNA methylation as an intermediary of genetic risk in rheumatoid arthritis. Nat Biotechnol 31:142–147

10. Houseman EA et al (2012) Open Access DNA methylation arrays as surrogate measures of cell mixture distribution. BMC Bioinformatics 13

11. Zou J et al (2014) Epigenome-wide association studies without the need for cell-type composition. Nat Methods 11:309–311

12. Lippert C et al (2011) FaST linear mixed models for genome-wide association studies. Nat Methods 8:833–835

13. Listgarten J et al (2012) Improved linear mixed models for genome-wide association studies. Nat Methods 9:525–526

14. Lippert C, Quon G, Listgarten J, Heckerman D (2013) The benefits of selecting phenotype-specific variants for applications of mixed models in genomics. Sci Rep 3:1815

15. Listgarten J, Lippert C, Heckerman D (2013) Fast-LMM-Select tackles confounding from spatial structure and rare variants. Nat Genet 45:470–471

16. Price AL et al (2006) Principal components analysis corrects for stratification in genome-wide association studies. Nat Genet 38:904–909

17. Leek JT, Storey JD (2007) Capturing heterogeneity in gene expression studies by surrogate variable analysis. PLoS Genet 3:1724–1735

Methods in Molecular Biology (2017) 1589: 115–138
DOI 10.1007/7651_2015_259
© Springer Science+Business Media New York 2015
Published online: 03 July 2016

Nano-MeDIP-seq Methylome Analysis Using Low DNA Concentrations

Lee M. Butcher and Stephan Beck

Abstract

DNA methylation is an epigenetic mark that is indispensable for mammalian development and occurs at cytosine residues throughout the genome (the "methylome"). Approximately 70 % of all CpG dinucleotides are affected by DNA methylation, which serve to "lock in" chromatin states and thus transcriptional programs. The systemic and pervasive occurrence of DNA methylation throughout the genome defines cellular identity and therefore requires genome-wide assays to fully appreciate and discern differential patterns of methylation that influence aspects of phenotypic plasticity including susceptibility to common complex disease.

One method that permits methylome analysis is methylated DNA immunoprecipitation (MeDIP) combined with next-generation sequencing (MeDIP-seq). MeDIP uses an antibody raised against 5-methylcytosine to capture methylated fragments of DNA, which are subsequently sequenced to envisage the methylome landscape. The advantageous cost versus coverage balance of MeDIP-seq has made it the method of choice to replace or complement array-based methods for population epigenetic studies. Here we detail nano-MeDIP-seq, which allows methylome analysis using nanogram quantities of starting material.

Keywords: Epigenetics, DNA methylation, Whole genome, Next-generation sequencing, Low concentration, Bioinformatics

1 Introduction

DNA methylation is the presence of a methyl group at the carbon-5 position of the cytosine pyrimidine ring, catalyzed by DNA methyltransferases [1] forming 5-methylcytosine. DNA methylation is present throughout the genome in a tissue- and cell-specific fashion, and its presence effectively "locks in" transcriptional programs dictated primarily by the local chromatin state. DNA methylation localizes to all inter- and intragenic features and, depending on where it occurs, can alter transcription both quantitatively (gene expression) and qualitatively (e.g., alternative splicing). There are a number of mechanisms by which DNA methylation achieves these effects and these are being discovered at an ever-increasing rate (*see* Ref. 2 for a review). The sequence context in which DNA methylation affects cytosines can be largely divided into two categories: at CG dinucleotides ("mCG") and non-CG dinucleotides ("mC"). Postimplantation, approximately 60–80 % (16.5–22.5 M) of CG dinucleotides are methylated in all nucleated human cells, including stem cell populations [3–5]. In embryonic pluripotent stem cells however, an additional 7.5 M cytosines are methylated at non-CG dinucleotides [3–5], which permits a myriad of additional regulatory controls to achieve diverse cellular phenotypes.

Given that DNA methylation is distributed genome wide, and that patterns of this distribution vary both within and between individuals for matched cell types, comprehensive and systematic assays are required. A number of technologies exist to meet this need (reviewed in ref. 6], including Methylated DNA immunoprecipitation or "MeDIP". MeDIP involves antibodies directed against mC or mCG to precipitate methylated DNA fragments. MeDIP is able to detect methylated cytosines in both mC and mCG contexts, and a major benefit is that it is capable of targeting the vast majority of the methylome.

Because antibodies used for MeDIP were raised in a way to yield equal specificity against mC and mCG, McDIP offers a hypothesis-free approach without prior assumptions about which regions of the methylome might be targeted. The most information-rich way of capitalizing on the largely balanced qualities of MeDIP has been to combine it with next-generation sequencing, or MeDIP-seq [7]. This application provides high-quality methylomes at typically 100- to 300-bp resolution (depending on chosen insert size) at costs comparable to other capture-based techniques [8] and was used to generate the first methylome of any mammalian genome [7].

One limitation of MeDIP-seq concerns genomic resolution. Although single-base pair resolution is desirable, we feel that the resolution offered by MeDIP-seq offsets issues of coverage and cost associated with single-base pair (e.g., bisulfite treatment) sequencing-oriented technologies. We also consider 150–200 bp to be a suitable resolution for most applications, as DNA methylation at adjacent CpGs is correlated for up to approximately 1 kb [9].

Another limitation of MeDIP-seq is that methylated DNA recovery by the antibody is affected by mC/mCG density, such that regions of very low (<1.5 %) density may be underrepresented or even interpreted as unmethylated. Furthermore, MeDIP enriches only for methylated portions of the genome, and unmethylated portions can only be inferred by an absence of reads. Consequently, the confidence placed on this inference is highly dependent on sequencing depth; the cost of this, however, is continually falling [10] and may cease to become a limiting factor in the future.

In addition to being a cost-effective method for analyzing all currently known forms of mammalian DNA methylation, the MeDIP-seq protocol has the advantage that as little as 50 ng DNA can be used [11]. This makes MeDIP-seq suitable for studies involving minute clinical samples, microdissected tissues, and rare cell types.

In our laboratory, MeDIP-seq libraries can be created in 3 days; however, inexperienced users might prefer to spread the protocol over 5 days. The time required for the actual sequencing depends on the model of the sequencer (at the time of writing an Illumina HiSeq 2500 takes ~5.5 days for a "high output" paired-end run of 50 bases). Bioinformatic processing, e.g., using MeDUSA [12] takes approximately 10 h.

2   Materials

2.1   Reagents

1. 1 M Tris–HCl (pH 7.8).

2. 1 M Tris–HCl (pH 8.0).

3. 1 M Tris–HCl (pH 8.5) [Elution buffer].

4. 0.5 M EDTA solution.

5. 5 M NaCl: Dissolve 292.2 g of NaCl in 1000 ml of PCR grade water. Store at room temperature and use within 2 years.

6. 1× sodium chloride-Tris–EDTA (STE) buffer: Mix 100 µl 1 M Tris–HCl (pH 7.8), 20 µl 0.5 M EDTA, and 100 µl 5 M NaCl in a total volume of 10 ml (fill up with PCR grade water). Store at room temperature and store indefinitely. Final concentrations: 10 mM Tris–HCl, 1 mM EDTA, and 50 mM NaCl.

7. 1× Tris–EDTA (TE) buffer: Mix 10 ml 1 M Tris–HCl (pH 8.0), 2 ml 0.5 M EDTA in a total volume of 1 l (fill up with PCR grade water). Store at room temperature and store indefinitely. Final concentrations: 10 mM Tris–HCl, 1 mM EDTA.

8. Lambda (λ)-DNA (NEB, cat. no. N3011S) for methylated control fragments.

9. SssI CpG methyltransferase (NEB, cat. no. M0226S).

10. Taq DNA Polymerase with 10× Buffer containing 25 mM $MgCl_2$ (ABgene, cat no. AB-0192/A).

11. Agencourt Ampure XP (60 ml; Beckman Coulter, cat. no. A63881).

12. Library Preparation End repair module (NEB, cat. no. E6050L).

13. Library Preparation A-tail module (NEB, cat. no. E6053L).

14. Library Preparation Adapter ligation module (NEB, cat. no. E6056L).

15. AutoMeDIP kit [Diagenode, cat. no. AF-Auto01-0016 (16 reactions) or AF-Auto01-0100 (100 reactions)] (*see* **Note 1**).

16. High-fidelity PCR kit (Kapa Biosystems, cat. no. KK2101).

17. Gel DNA Recovery Kit (Zymo Research, cat. no. D4001).

18. 96–100 % Ethanol.

19. 70 % Ethanol.

20. Agarose.

21. 50 bp DNA Ladder (*see* **Note 2**).

22. 10× Tris–Borate EDTA (TBE).

23. Ethidium bromide (10 mg/ml).

24. Gel loading dye containing bromophenol blue, xylene cyanol, and orange G.

25. DNA1000 kit (Agilent, cat. no. 5067-1504).

26. High Sensitivity kit (Agilent, cat. no. 5067-4626).

27. SYBR qPCR master mix.

28. PCR grade water.

29. Paired-end (PE) sequencing adapters (*see* **Note 3**). Spin down lyophilized adapter oligos in a chilled (4 °C) microcentrifuge at $200 \times g$ for 5 min. Resuspend each oligo in 1× STE buffer to 100 μM. Add equimolar quantities of each adapter into a 1.5 ml microcentrifuge tube. Divide into small (e.g., 200 μl) aliquots and incubate at 95 °C for 15 min, and then leave to cool down to room temperature (~1 h). Store aliquots at −20 °C until required. Final concentration: 50 μM.

30. Adapter-mediated PCR primers (*see* **Note 4**). Spin down lyophilized primer oligos in a chilled (4 °C) microcentrifuge at $200 \times g$ for 5 min. Resuspend each oligo in Elution buffer to create 100 μM stocks. Dilute aliquots tenfold in 1 × TE buffer to create 10 μM dilutions. Store dilutions in manageable volumes at −20 °C until required.

31. Quality Control (QC) primers (*see* **Note 5**).

2.2 Equipment

1. Microcentrifuge tubes (0.5, 1.5, and 2 ml).

2. 8-strip, 0.2 ml PCR tubes and caps.

3. 12-strip, 0.2 ml PCR tubes and caps.

4. IP-Star tips (Diagenode, cat. no. WC-001-1000).

5. qPCR plates and seals.

6. Centrifuge with 0.2 ml tube adapter ("microfuge").

7. Centrifuge with 2.0 ml adaptors.

8. Pipettes.

9. Pipette filter tips.

10. Vortex.

11. Transilluminator and imaging software.

12. Microwave oven.

13. Magnetic separation rack.

14. Scalpels.

15. Thermocycler.

16. qPCR system.

17. Gel electrophoresis system (inc. gel tanks and combs).

18. Weighing scale and weighing boats.

19. Sonicator (*see* **Note 6**).

20. Heat block or oven.

21. Agilent Bioanalyzer 2100.

22. Illumina sequencer (*see* **Note 7**).

23. SX-8G IP-Star (*see* **Note 8**).

3 Methods

Before creating MeDIP-seq libraries, it is worth spending time familiarizing oneself with the workflow (*see* Fig. 1).

3.1 Creation of Methylated and Unmethylated Controls

The following describes a one-off set of procedures to create a central laboratory resource of methylated and unmethylated control fragments that should be suitable for over a million MeDIP assays.

1. For each control region, combine the following reagents in a 0.2 ml PCR tube (note, it is often more convenient to make a mastermix excluding primers):

Reagent	×1 reaction (μl)
10× Reaction buffer IV	2.5
MgCl$_2$ (25 mM)	1.0
dNTP mix (10 mM)	1.0
Forward primer (*see* Table 1)	1.25
Reverse primer (*see* Table 1)	1.25
PCR grade water	17.625
λ-DNA (0.0005 ng/μl)	1.0
Taq DNA polymerase	0.125
Total volume/reaction	25.0

2. Pipette mix and briefly centrifuge in a microfuge to consolidate reactions.

MeDIP-seq workflow

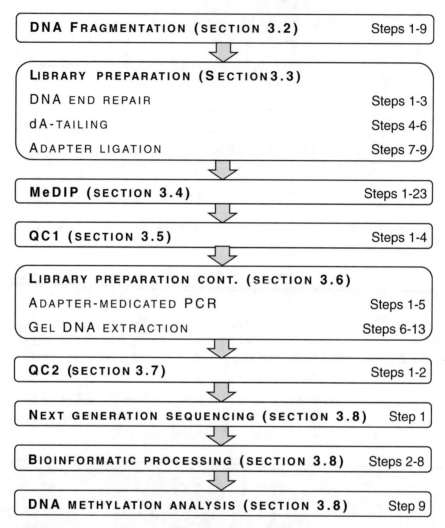

Fig. 1 The MeDIP-seq workflow. MeDIP-seq libraries can be created in 3 days. The time required for the actual sequencing depends on the model of the sequencer (at the time of writing, an Illumina HiSeq 2500 takes ~5.5 days for a "high output" paired-end run of 50 bases). Bioinformatic processing takes approximately 10 h

3. Set up and run the following PCR program: incubate for 2 min at 94 °C, followed by a total of 40 cycles of (20 s at 94 °C, 30 s with touchdown: 53/65 °C, 60 s at 72 °C), then 5 min at 72 °C.

4. Purify amplicons using 1.8 volumes Ampure XP purification beads according to manufacturer's procedure (*see* **Note 9**) and elute in 10 µl Elution buffer.

5. Run the sample on an Agilent Bioanalyzer 2100 using DNA1000 chips and reagents according to manufacturer's

Table 1
Details of the oligos used in the protocol. CpG% is defined as $2 \times$ number CpGs/fragment length [bp]. For fragments derived from the fragmented sample DNA, CpG% was estimated by simulation. Enterobacteria phage lambda genomic Start and Stop coordinates were derived from accession number NC_001416; human genomic start and stop coordinates were derived from reference assembly GRCh37.p2; mouse genomic start and stop coordinates were derived from reference assembly MGSCv37

Oligo name	Genome	Sequence (5' → 3')	Length (bp)	CpG (%)	Amplicon size (bp)	Start	End
Adapter PE 1.0[a]	N/A	[Phos]GATCGGAAGAGCGGTT CAGCAGGAATGCCGAG	33	N/A	N/A	N/A	N/A
Adapter PE 2.0[a]	N/A	ACACTCTTTCCCTACACGAC GCTCTTCCGATC*T	32	N/A	N/A	N/A	N/A
Adapter InPE 1.0[b]	N/A	[Phos]GATCGGAAGAGCACAC GTCT	20	N/A	N/A	N/A	N/A
Adapter InPE 2.0[b]	N/A	ACACTCTTTCCCTACACGACG CTCTTCCGATC*T	33	N/A	N/A	N/A	N/A
PCR.primer.PE.1.0 (F)[a]	N/A	AATGATACGGCGACCACCGAG ATCTACACTCTTTCCCTACA CGACGCTCTTCCGATC*T	58	N/A	N/A	N/A	N/A
PCR.primer.PE.2.0 (R)[a]	N/A	CAAGCAGAAGACGGCATACG AGATCGGTCTCGGCATTC CTGCTGAACCGCTCTTCCGATC*T	61	N/A	N/A	N/A	N/A
PCR primer InPE 1.0 (F)[b]	N/A	AATGATACGGCGACCACCGA GATCTACACTCTTTCCCTA CACGACGCTCTTCCGATC*T	58	N/A	N/A	N/A	N/A
PCR primer InPE 2.1 (R)[b]	N/A	CAAGCAGAAGACGGCATACG AGATCGTGATGTGACTGGA GTTCAGACGTGTGCTCTTCCGATC*T	64	N/A	N/A	N/A	N/A
PCR primer InPE 2.2 (R)[b]	N/A	CAAGCAGAAGACGGCATACG AGATACATCGGTGACTGG AGTTCAGACGTGTGCTCTTCCGATC*T	64	N/A	N/A	N/A	N/A
PCR primer InPE 2.3 (R)[b]	N/A	CAAGCAGAAGACGGCATACG AGATGCCTAAGTGACTGGA GTTCAGACGTGTGCTCTTCCGATC*T	64	N/A	N/A	N/A	N/A
PCR primer InPE 2.4 (R)[b]	N/A	CAAGCAGAAGACGGCATACG AGATTGGTCAGTGACTGGA GTTCAGACGTGTGCTCTTCCGATC*T	64	N/A	N/A	N/A	N/A

(continued)

Table 1
(continued)

Oligo name	Genome	Sequence (5′ → 3′)	Length (bp)	CpG (%)	Amplicon size (bp)	Start	End
PCR primer InPE 2.5 (R)[b]	N/A	CAAGCAGAAGACGGCATACG AGATCACTGTGTGACTGGA GTTCAGACGTGTGCTCTTCCGATC*T	64	N/A	N/A	N/A	N/A
PCR primer InPE 2.6 (R)[b]	N/A	CAAGCAGAAGACGGCATA CGAGATATTGGCGTGACT GGAGTTCAGACGTGTGC TCTTCCGATC*T	64	N/A	N/A	N/A	N/A
PCR primer InPE 2.7 (R)[b]	N/A	CAAGCAGAAGACGGCATACG AGATGATCTGGTGACTGG AGTTCAGACGTGTGCTCTTCCGATC*T	64	N/A	N/A	N/A	N/A
PCR primer InPE 2.8 (R)[b]	N/A	CAAGCAGAAGACGGCATACG AGATTCAAGTGTGACTGG AGTTCAGACGTGTGCTCTTCCGATC*T	64	N/A	N/A	N/A	N/A
PCR primer InPE 2.9 (R)[b]	N/A	CAAGCAGAAGACGGCATA CGAGATCTGATCGTGA CTGGAGTTCAGACGTG TGCTCTTCCGATC*T	64	N/A	N/A	N/A	N/A
PCR primer InPE 2.10 (R)[b]	N/A	CAAGCAGAAGACGGCATA CGAGATAAGCTAGTGA CTGGAGTTCAGACGTG TGCTCTTCCGATC*T	64	N/A	N/A	N/A	N/A
PCR primer InPE 2.11 (R)[b]	N/A	CAAGCAGAAGACGGCAT ACGAGATGTAGCCGT GACTGGAGTTCAGAC GTGTGCTCTTCCGATC*T	64	N/A	N/A	N/A	N/A
PCR primer InPE 2.12 (R)[b]	N/A	CAAGCAGAAGACGGCATACG AGATTACAAGGTGACTGG AGTTCAGACGTGTGCTCT TCCGATC*T	64	N/A	N/A	N/A	N/A

Primer	Template	Sequence	Length				
1CpG_qPCR_F	λ-DNA	ACAAGTTGTTGATCTTTGC	20	N/A	145	24004	24148
1CpG_qPCR_R		CCTATGAGCAACGTGTTAG	19				
5CpG_qPCR_F		CACTTGAATCTGTGGTTCAT	20	N/A	130	25942	26071
5CpG_qPCR_R		TAGAAAAGACAACTCTGGC	20				
10CpG_qPCR_F		GAACTCACACAACACCA	19	N/A	125	33662	33786
10CpG_qPCR_R		ACTCTGAATACCGACTCAAT	20				
15CpG_qPCR_F		TATCACTGTTGATTCTGC	19	N/A	121	28669	28789
15CpG_qPCR_R		GGTAAAGAGTTTGGATTAGG	20				
20CpG_L_qPCR_F		GGTGAACTTCCGATAGTG	18	N/A	108	24202	24309
20CpG_L_qPCR_R		CAGTCATAGATGGTCGGT	18				
20CpG_S_qPCR_F		GTTAGAGCCTGCATAACG	18	N/A	109	44747	44855
20CpG_S_qPCR_R		GAAAGAGCACTGGCTAAC	18				
1CpG_F		GAGGTGATAAAATTAACTGC	20	0.5	197	23967	24163
1CpG_R		GGCTCTACCATATCTCCTA	19				
5CpG_F		CATGTCCAGAGCTCATTC	18	4.0	270	25869	26138
5CpG_R		GTTTAAAATCACTAGGCGA	19				
10CpG_F		CTGACCATTCCATCATTC	19	5.6	360	33638	33997
10CpG_R		GTAACTAAACAGGAGCCG	18				
15CpG_F		ATGTATCCATTGAGCATTGCC	21	6.4	462	28488	28949
15CpG_R		CACGAATCAGCGGTAAAGGT	20				
20CpG_L_F		GAGATATGGTAGAGCGCAGA	21	8.0	275	24148	24643
20CpG_L_R		TTTCAGCAGCTACAGTCAGAATTT	24				
20CpG_S_F		CGATGGGTTAATTCGCTCGTTGTGG	25	14.6	403	44589	44863
20CpG_S_R		GCACAACGGAAAGAGCACTG	20				
MM_meth_qPCR_F	Mouse	CATGGCCCACAAAGTAATAAAA	22	16.0	93	Chr1:19718938	Chr1:19719030
MM_meth_qPCR_R		AACGACTTACAACGAGCTCAAA	22				
MM_unme_qPCR_F		GGCTAGAACTGACCAGACAGAC	22	16.0	86	Chr4:16751777	Chr4:16751862
MM_unme_qPCR_R		ATCTGTAGCCAATCCTAGAGCA	22				
HS_meth_qPCR_F	Human	GGGAATATAAGGAGCGCACA	18	10.0	114	Chr22:29607176	Chr22:29607289
HS_meth_qPCR_R		TCGGTTAAAACGGTCAGGTC	18				
HS_unme_qPCR_F		CGAGGCGTGAGTTATTCCTG	20	10.0	110	Ch6:4011057	Chr6:4011166
HS_unme_qPCR_R		CTCTTGTGGCTGAGCTCCTT	20				

[*] = phosphorothioate; [Phos] = 3′-phosphate
[a]Adapters and amPCR primers for single-plex library prep
[b]Adapters and amPCR primers for multiplex library prep

instructions. Verify DNA fragment size range and concentration using the instrument's software.

6. Divide each amplicon into two aliquots and label.

7. Set up one in vitro methylation reaction and one control reaction for each aliquot in a 0.2 ml PCR tube as follows and incubate for 2 h at 37 °C, followed by 20 min at 65 °C:

Reagent	In vitro methylation reaction (μl)	Control reaction (μl)
PCR grade water	10.0	11.0
10× NEBuffer 2	2.0	2.0
S-adenosylmethionine (1.6 mM)	2.0	2.0
Amplicon DNA (from **step 4**)	5.0	5.0
SssI methyltransferase (4 U/μl)	1.0	–
Total volume/reaction	20.0	20.0

8. Purify each reaction using 1.8 volumes Ampure XP purification beads according to manufacturer's procedure and elute in 10 μl Elution buffer.

9. Each amplicon contains at least one 5′-ACGT-3′ motif, which allows the methylation status of each region to be verified using the methylation sensitive enzyme, *HpyCH4*IV. To do so, dilute 1 μl of each amplicon from each reaction 1 in 10 with PCR grade water.

10. Set up the following reaction for each diluted DNA incubate for 1 h at 37 °C then 20 min at 65 °C:

Reagent	×1 reaction (μl)
10× NEBuffer 1	2.5
*HpyCH4*IV (10 U/μl)	1.0
Diluted DNA	10
PCR grade water	11.5
Total volume/reaction	25.0

11. Purify each sample using 1.8 volumes Ampure XP purification beads according to manufacturer's procedure and elute in 10 μl Elution buffer.

12. Run the sample on an Agilent Bioanalyzer 2100 using DNA1000 chips and reagents according to manufacturer's instructions. Validate DNA fragment size range and concentration using the instrument's software (*see* **Note 10**).

13. Create 1 nM working dilutions of methylated and unmethylated controls based on Bioanalyzer readings

14. Use the 1 nM dilutions to create a equimolar cocktail of control fragments consisting of methylated (0.5, 3.7, 5.6, 6.5, and 10 % CpG density) and unmethylated (14.5 % CpG density) fragments.

15. Store stock solutions and working dilutions (e.g., 10 µM) of in vitro methylated and unmethylated fragments at −20 °C indefinitely

16. Run the sample on an Agilent Bioanalyzer 2100 using DNA High Sensitivity chips and reagents according to manufacturer's instructions. Validate DNA fragment size range and concentration using the instrument's software (*see* **Note 11**).

17. Dilute the cocktail in 1 × TE buffer to create a 100 pM (each) stock cocktail.

18. Dilute aliquots of the 100 pM stock in 1× TE buffer to create working dilutions of 0.19 pM (or ~114,000 copies per µl) (*see* **Note 12**).

3.2 DNA Fragmentation

1. In a 0.5 or 1.5 ml microcentrifuge tube, resuspend gDNA in 85 µl Elution buffer.

2. Pre-chill the sonicator water bath by filling with ice and leave for 15 min.

3. After 15 min, replace the ice in the water bath with ice-cold water.

4. Place microcentrifuge tube containing DNA in the appropriate tube holder, making sure the holder is balanced.

5. Set sonicator to "High" and sonicate for 15 min consisting of 30-s on/off periods.

6. Following 15 min cycle, briefly centrifuge DNA samples and store on ice.

7. Cool the sonicator for 5–10 min by filling with crushed ice.

8. Repeat **steps 5–7** up to another six times (*see* **Note 13**).

9. Run the sample on an Agilent Bioanalyzer 2100 using High Sensitivity DNA chips and reagents according to manufacturer's instructions; validate DNA fragment size range and concentration using the instrument's software (*see* **Note 14**).

3.3 Library Preparation (1 of 2)

1. *DNA end repair*: Mix the following on ice in a sterile PCR tube and incubate for 30 min at 20 °C. Scale accordingly.

Reagent	×1 reaction (μl)
NEBNext end repair enzyme mix	5
NEBNext end repair reaction buffer (10×)	10
Fragmented DNA	85
Total volume	100

2. Place the reaction on ice after incubation, spin briefly in a microfuge for ~3 s to collect condensate.

3. Purify DNA sample using 1.8 volumes Ampure XP purification beads according to manufacturer's procedure and elute in 37 μl Elution buffer.

4. *dA-tailing*. Mix the following on ice in a sterile PCR tube and incubate for 30 min at 37 °C (*see* **Note 15**). Scale accordingly.

Reagent	×1 reaction (μl)
Klenow fragment (3′ → 5′ exo⁻)	3
NEBNext dA-tailing reaction buffer (10×)	5
PCR grade water	5
Purified end-repaired, blunt-ended DNA from step 3	37
Total volume	50

5. Purify DNA sample using 1.8 volumes Ampure XP purification beads according to manufacturer's procedure and elute in 25 μl Elution buffer.

6. Calculate the reaction concentration of DNA adapters to be used in the adapter ligation reaction (*see* **Note 16**).

7. *Adapter ligation*. Mix the following on ice in a sterile PCR tube and incubate in a thermocycler for 2 h at 18 °C. Scale accordingly.

Reagent	×1 Reaction (μl)
Quick ligation reaction buffer (5×)	10
Adapters	*Variable*
PCR grade water to 50 μl	*As required*
End-repaired, blunt, dA-tailed DNA from step 5	25
Quick T4 DNA ligase	5
Total volume	50

8. Purify DNA sample using 1.8 volumes Ampure XP purification beads according to manufacturer's procedure and elute in 40 μl Elution buffer.

9. Run 1 μl of eluted sample on an Agilent Bioanalyzer 2100 using High Sensitivity DNA chips and reagents according to manufacturer's instructions; determine the concentration of the full range of DNA fragments (*see* **Note 17**).

3.4 Methylated DNA Immunoprecipitation

1. Perform MeDIP on purified adapter-ligated DNA from step 8 (previous section), using the Diagenode AutoMeDIP and SX-8G IP-star (*see* **Notes 1** and **18**).

2. *Antibody (Ab) Dilution.* Mix the following on ice and scale accordingly (see next step):

Reagent	Vol (μl)
Antibody	1
PCR grade water	15
Total volume	16

3. *Antibody Mix.* Mix the following on ice:

Reagent	×1 IP (μl)
Diluted Ab (from step 2)	2.40
MagBuffer A (5×)	0.60
MagBuffer C	2.00
Total volume	5.00

4. *1 × Magbuffer A.* Gently mix the following on ice and scale accordingly:

Reagent	×1 IP (μl)
MagBuffer A (5×)	30
PCR grade water	120
Total volume	150

5. *Incubation Mix.* Mix the following (sufficient for 1 × IP and 1 × Input) on ice and scale accordingly:

Reagent	×1 IP
MagBuffer A (5×)	24 μl
MagBuffer B	6 μl
Lambda Spike cocktail (0.2 pM each; *see* **Note 1**)	3 μl
Purified adapter-ligated DNA	*Variable*
PCR grade water up to 90 μl	*As required*
Total volume/reaction	90 μl

6. Incubate *Incubation Mix(es)* at 99 °C for 10 min.

7. Snap cool on ice for 10 min.

8. Switch on the IP-Star (*see* **Note 19**).

9. Mix the *Incubation Mix(es)* by pipetting up and down and spin for 3 s on microfuge.

   The following steps detail the loading of the IP-Star (a description of the automated process is presented in **Note 20**).

10. Load reagents into a 12-strip tube as per Fig. 2 (one strip tube per IP).

11. Place the filled 12-strip on the Peltier block(s) (*see* Fig. 3, black-boxed zone and **Notes 21–23**).

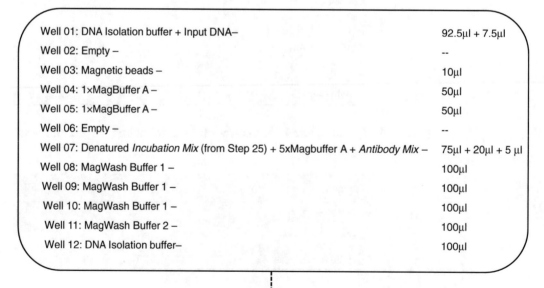

Well 01: DNA Isolation buffer + Input DNA–	92.5μl + 7.5μl
Well 02: Empty –	--
Well 03: Magnetic beads –	10μl
Well 04: 1×MagBuffer A –	50μl
Well 05: 1×MagBuffer A –	50μl
Well 06: Empty –	--
Well 07: Denatured *Incubation Mix* (from Step 25) + 5xMagbuffer A + *Antibody Mix* –	75μl + 20μl + 5 μl
Well 08: MagWash Buffer 1 –	100μl
Well 09: MagWash Buffer 1 –	100μl
Well 10: MagWash Buffer 1 –	100μl
Well 11: MagWash Buffer 2 –	100μl
Well 12: DNA Isolation buffer–	100μl

Well: 01 02 03 04 05 06 07 08 09 10 11 12

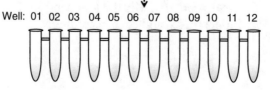

Fig. 2 Reaction mixes for a single AutoMeDIP run. Reagents are mixed and dispensed into 12-strip tubes prior to starting an AutoMeDIP run, at which point the IP-Star performs MeDIP sequentially across the wells

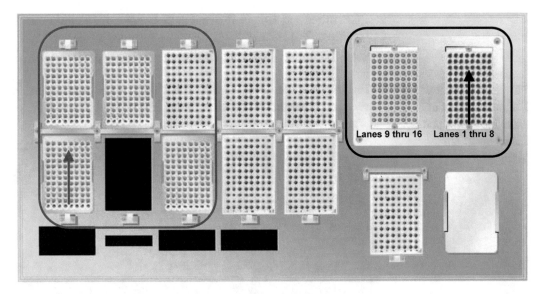

Fig. 3 Layout of the IP-Star bed. The *red-boxed zone* illustrates the location of tip holders; the *black-boxed zone* shows the two 96-well Peltier blocks. The *arrows* demonstrate the direction of workflow of the IP-Star. Twelve consecutive wells are called "lanes"; when ≤ 8 IPs are being performed, only the right Peltier block (*lanes 1–8*) is used; when >8 IPs are being performed, both blocks are used. It is important to match tips in lanes of tip racks with samples in lanes of Peltier blocks

12. Place IP-Star tips into tip rack (*see* Fig. 3, red-boxed zone; *see* **Note 24**).

13. Double click a tip rack in the GUI until it shows tips are present. The clicked tip rack should correspond to the tip rack just filled.

14. Select **8IPs or 16IPs** protocol for 8 and 16 MeDIP reactions respectively.

15. Click "Modify" to set IP incubation time and temperature (*see* **Note 25**).

16. Press *Start* and OK the confirmation screen that appears: The automated MeDIP reaction starts. After the IP-Star has eluted the mDNA-Ab-bead complex in DIB solution, a dialog box appears on the screen.

17. Add 1 μl proteinase K (from AutoMeDIP kit) to well 1 and well 12 for each 12-strip.

18. Add 7.5 μl Input DNA into well 1 of the 12-strip.

19. Cap the 12-strip.

20. OK the dialog box and close the IP-Star door.

21. OK the dialog box; the proteinase K digestion reaction will start.

22. Once completed, a confirmation message appears in the GUI: Remove samples from the IP-Star and transfer the contents of well 12 (proteinase K digested IP reaction) into clean 0.2 ml

PCR tubes and collect the magnetic beads on a magnetic rack (*see* **Note 26**).

23. Shut down the IP-Star software and turn off the IP-Star off.

3.5 Quality Control: Test for Recovery of Spiked-in λ-DNA and Specificity of the MeDIP Reaction (QC 1)

1. Prepare the following on ice in a qPCR plate: perform each reaction in triplicate for methylated and unmethylated control regions (*see* Table 1).

Reagent	×1 reaction (μl)
2× SYBR qPCR master mix	6.25
Primer pair (10 μM)	0.625
PCR grade water	4.375
MeDIP or input DNA (from step 22 of previous section)	1.25
Total volume/reaction	12.5

2. Seal plate and centrifuge briefly to ensure no bubbles remain at the bottom the wells.

3. Run the following program on a real time PCR machine: (1) 95 °C for 5 min, (2) 40 cycles of 95 °C for 15 s, 60 °C for 1 min, (3) melt curve.

4. Calculate Recovery and Specificity (*see* **Note 27**).

For troubleshooting problems associated with the MeDIP reaction, *see* Table 2.

3.6 Library Preparation (2 of 2)

1. Purify DNA sample (from step 22 of Section 3.4) using 1.8 volumes Ampure XP purification beads according to manufacturer's procedure and elute in 25 μl Elution buffer.

2. *Adapter-mediated PCR (amPCR)*. On ice, mix and scale accordingly the following in a sterile PCR tube. Pipette up and down to mix.

Reagent	×1 reaction (μl)
5× KAPA GC buffer	10
10 mM dNTP mix	1.5
Forward primer (10 μM)	5
Reverse primer (10 μM)	5
DMSO	2.5
Purified MeDIP DNA (from step 1)	25
KAPA HiFi polymerase (1 U/μl)	1
Total volume	50

Table 2
Troubleshooting guide

Step	Problem	Possible reason	Solution
3.5	No recovery of MeDIP fraction	IP incubation time too short	Increase IP incubation time
		Ab AND/OR beads	Check all reagents have been correctly dispensed
		Poor construction of control cocktail	Check control cocktail sequences are methylated using methylation-specific enzyme
			Check control cocktail sequences amplify independently of MeDIP-seq experiment
			Try using species-specific qPCR primers to validate recovery of MeDIP (expect 10–20 % recovery)
		None of the above?	Repeat MeDIP on adapter-ligated DNA
	Low (<10 %) recovery of MeDIP fraction and low (<90 %) specificity	IP incubation time too short	Increase IP incubation time
		Aspiration of bead complex following IP (manual only)	If beads remain in tips between MeDIP and purification, pipette mix the solution until no beads remain in the tip
		None of the above?	Repeat MeDIP on adapter-ligated DNA
	Low (<10 %) recovery but high (>95 %) specificity	IP incubation time too short but MeDIP should not be considered failed	Proceed to amPCR (step 41) and evaluate
	Ct values for both QC regions in MeDIP fraction are similar	IP Incubation temperature too high	Reduce IP incubation temperature to 4 °C
		Incorrect PCR product has been amplified	Check qPCR melt curve
3.6	No or very low post-amPCR yield	Poor or very inefficient adapter ligation	Check that peak size (assessed using Bioanalyzer) of fragments increases between sonication and adapter ligation
			Dilute post-adapter-ligated samples 1 in 10 and perform a single amPCR reaction; should see a smear on a gel

(continued)

Table 2
(continued)

Step	Problem	Possible reason	Solution
			Ensure samples have been purified prior to amPCR
3.7	Little or no enrichment of methylated regions in MeDIP fraction	PCR failure	Check gel for DNA smear
		Gel purification failure	Ensure adequate volumes of Buffer QG are used
			Ensure pH of QG & sample is at correct pH (<7.5); if not add 10 μl 3 M NaAc (pH 5.0)
		Inaccurate DNA quantification	Use agilent high sensitivity DNA chips. Avoid spectrophotometry
		MeDIP and input sample concentrations not normalized	Normalize MeDIP and input sample concentrations to >0.1 ng/μl
		Poor starting DNA quality	Ensure approximately 25–30 % of starting DNA falls into the desired excision range
3.8	Low proportion of aligned reads	Low quality base score at 3′ end of read	Trim bases from the sequence prior to alignment

3. Split each reaction into two 25 μl aliquots and perform PCR in a preheated thermocycler, using the following cycling conditions: (1) 95 °C for 2 min, (2) 8–13 cycles of: 98 °C for 20 s, 60 °C for 15 s, 72 °C for 15 s, (3) 72 °C for 5 min.

4. Combine the two PCR MeDIP reactions and purify DNA sample with 1.8 volumes Ampure XP purification beads and elute in 15 μl Elution buffer (*see* **Note 28**).

5. Run 1 μl of eluted sample on an Agilent Bioanalyzer 2100 using DNA1000 chips and reagents according to manufacturer's instructions; validate DNA fragment size range using the instrument's software. For troubleshooting *see* Table 2.

6. Prepare a 2 % TBE agarose gel, with 0.5 μl/ml Ethidium Bromide (*see* **Note 29**).

7. Mix the remaining PCR amplified MeDIP reactions (from step 4) with an appropriate volume of loading dye and load on gel, leaving space either side for ladders (*see* **Note 29**).

8. Load 1 μg of a 50 bp DNA ladder in wells flanking the DNA sample.

9. Carry out gel electrophoresis in freshly prepared 1× TBE buffer at 100 V until orange G dye runs off gel.

10. Following gel electrophoresis, carefully transfer gel onto a UV transilluminator.

11. With a clean scalpel, excise the desired 50 bp library size range (*see* **Note 30**). Ensure the gel slice is cut as close to DNA smear as possible (*see* **Notes 31** and **32**).

12. Purify DNA libraries using Gel DNA Recovery Kit (Zymo Research) according to manufacturer's protocol and elute in 10 μl Elution buffer.

13. Assess 1 μl of size selected DNA on an Agilent Bioanalyzer using High Sensitivity DNA chips and reagents according to manufacturer's instructions to determine gel extraction has worked.

3.7 Quality Control: Test for Enrichment of Methylated Regions (QC 2)

1. Dilute 1 μl of size selected DNA to 9 μl with PCR grade water and validate the enrichment of genomic regions of known methylation status (*see* Table 1 and **Note 5**) by qPCR using reaction setup as detailed in steps 1 and 2 of Section 3.6.

2. Calculate enrichment as described in **Note 33**. For troubleshooting *see* Table 2.

3.8 Next-Generation Sequencing and Bioinformatic Processing

1. Subject sample to next-generation sequencing with an Illumina machine that uses flowcells compatible with the primer sequences used during amPCR according to manufacturer's instructions.

2. Use FastQC (http://www.bioinformatics.bbsrc.ac.uk/projects/fastqc/) to perform quality control of the reads.

3. Align MeDIP-seq reads to the relevant reference genome using BWA (*see* **Note 34**).

4. Use BWA to run "bwa aln" on both read ends to generate two .sai output files.

5. Use BWA to run "bwa sampe" using the .sai files from previous step as input; the output is a SAM formatted alignment file.

6. Use SAMtools to discard reads from the SAM formatted alignment file that fail to map as a proper pair.

7. Use MeDUSA to discard read pairs in which neither read scored a BWA alignment score ≥10.

8. Use MeDUSA to identify groups of nonunique reads (i.e., "clonal reads"—reads that align to the exact same start and stop position on the same chromosome) to discard all but one read from the group.

9. Perform MeDIP-seq specific QC on the filtered data from previous step using MeDIPs.

4 Notes

1. MeDIP can also be performed manually using, e.g., the Mag-MeDIP kit (Diagenode, cat. no. mc-magme-A10) or other kits/reagents. In this case, we advise taking care with respect to accurate and consistent timing of incubation steps, as well as performing lengthy and thorough bead washing steps.

2. To increase the accuracy of gel excision, we advise using a ladder with molecular-weight standards ranging from 50 to 700 bp in 50-bp size intervals.

3. Depending on the experimental design, single-plex or multi-plex Illumina adapters can be created and ligated to fragmented DNA. Table 1 presents adapter sequences for single-plex and multiplex applications, although other adapter systems could be used (e.g., see seqanswers.com) provided they DO NOT contain methylated cytosines.

4. Depending on the experimental design (e.g., single-plex or multiplex library construction), primers complementary to the appropriate Illumina adapters should be used. Table 1 presents primer sequences for single-plex and multiplex applications, although other primers compatible with other adapter systems can be used (e.g., see seqanswers.com). If multiplexing, always pool >3 indexed samples for sequencing.

5. For QC1, nested qPCR primers were designed for each λ-DNA fragment; sequences are presented in Table 1. For QC2, primers were designed to amplify regions of assumed methylation status in appropriate reference genomes, e.g., for previous work in humans *see* Ref. 13; we present example sequences for mouse and human in Table 1. Prepare and treat oligos as detailed in **Note 5**.

6. We recommend using the Bioruptor (Diagenode) sonicator for DNA fragmentation; however, other methods can be applied provided these can generate the specified DNA fragment range and peak.

7. The protocol detailed in these pages describes applications compatible with MiSeq, GAIIx, and HiSeq instruments.

8. We use the SX-8G IP-Star for our automated MeDIP-seq protocol, as it was specially designed and programmed for this purpose; however, generic liquid handlers can be programmed to carry out the MeDIP step as detailed in the MagMeDIP protocol (Diagenode).

9. After the second ethanol wash, keep the tubes on the magnetic rack and heat in an oven at 55 °C for about 7 min to evaporate all the ethanol. When the bead pellet starts to crack, this is a good time to elute.

10. In vitro methylated fragments will not be digested by HpyCH4IV and will result in intact, full-length fragments that correspond to the length of the original amplicon; unmethylated fragments will be digested at the restriction site and show multiple fragment lengths.

11. The molarity of each fragment in the cocktail is expected to be 166 pM. If not, correct accordingly by adding more of the required fragment(s) to normalize concentrations and recheck on a Bioanalyzer 2100 with High Sensitivity chips.

12. For the vast majority of QC purposes, we find that qPCR of just two regions [one methylated (10 % CpG density) and one unmethylated (14 % CpG density)] is sufficient to evaluate MeDIP. However, the full range of fragments in the cocktail can be assayed if desired.

13. Fragmented DNA can be stored at −20 °C for up to 1 month.

14. We aim to fragment the sample so the majority of fragments are below 500 bp and that 25–30 % of fragments are between 150 and 250 bp.

15. If using a thermocycler, use a heated lid (100 °C) during all incubations involving temperatures over 30 °C to prevent evaporation of samples.

16. To achieve tenfold excess molarity of adapters to DNA fragments in a 50 μl reaction, the following heuristic provides a good estimate:

$$\text{adapters}_{\text{rxn\_conc}}(\text{nM}) = \frac{606.1 \times r^2 \times \text{ng}}{\text{bp}},$$

where ng is starting concentration of DNA, bp is average size of DNA fragments, and r is estimated recovery from beads. For example, a starting concentration of 200 ng DNA with average size of 180 bp, assuming 0.8 (80 %) recovery from beads, will require a reaction concentration of adapters of approximately 431 nM.

17. If multiple samples are being run, determine the concentration across a set size range of fragments (e.g., 240–290 bp) using the "Smear Analysis" feature of the Bioanalyzer software. Sample input (ng) can then be normalized across samples during MeDIP to maintain reaction stoichiometry.

18. The following six steps deviate from the manufacturer's instruction and represent optimized steps.

19. The IP-Star takes approximately 10 min to equilibrate to the appropriate temperature (4 °C), so now is a convenient time to switch it on.

20. The IP-Star (Diagenode) is capable of automating up to 16 MeDIPs per run. Each run is split into two parts with a manual intervention step in between. In the first part, the IP-Star washes the magnetic beads (to remove any preservatives), immunoselects and captures the methylated fraction, washes away unbound (unmethylated) DNA and elutes in a proteinase K buffer. The second part requires the manual addition of input DNA well 1 and proteinase K to wells 1 and 12; this is followed by two 15 min incubations at 55 and 95 °C, respectively; the Peltier block then cools to 4 °C until the user removes the samples. A small proportion of these products are subject to quality control by qPCR (see below) and the rest are purified. The result is a pure, methylated fraction ready for amPCR.

21. Peltier blocks and tip racks of the IP-Star should be conceptualized as 96-well plates, i.e., 90° clockwise to the user. We call a row of 12 wells a "lane" and the MeDIP protocol proceeds in the direction of the arrow so align Well 1 of the 12-strip tube with the beginning of the arrow.

22. If running 8 or fewer IPs, load the 12-strips in the right-hand Peltier block. If running >8 IPs, load the remaining 12-strips in the left-hand Peltier block.

23. If running >8 IPs, it is best to balance the workload across both Peltier blocks and mirror the layout between blocks. Therefore, if running an odd number of IPs >8, we recommend placing an empty 12-strip on the Peltier block containing fewer samples, to mirror the formation of the Peltier block with more samples.

24. Each IP lane in the Peltier Block should have a corresponding lane of IP-Star tips in a tip rack. When performing eight or fewer IPs, load 6 IP-Star tips per lane; if performing between 8 and 16 IPs, load 9 IP-Star tips per lane. Tip lanes must correspond to sample lanes.

25. IP incubation times are for each block. We recommend at least 7.5 h incubation time (15 h is preferable) and 4 °C incubation temperature

26. MeDIP and Input DNA can be stored at −20 °C for up to 3 months and longer at −80 °C

27. From the qPCR results, "Recovery" and "Specificity" are calculated to evaluate MeDIP efficiency. Recovery, which is a measure of the MeDIP efficiency—indexed as percentage input—is calculated using the cycle threshold (Ct) of MeDIP and Input fractions from the qPCR reaction. Since only 10 % of the DNA used in MeDIP is used for Input, the Ct value

obtained for the Input is adjusted prior to calculating Recovery, using the formula:

$$\text{Adjusted Input Ct} = \text{Input Ct} - \frac{\log_{10}(10)}{\log_{10}(2 \times \text{AE})}$$

where AE is the % amplification efficiency expressed as a decimal (e.g., 100 % AE = 1) and 10 represents the dilution factor of Input to MeDIP (i.e., 75 μl IP vs. 7.5 μl Input = ×10).

Recovery is then calculated for each set of primers as:

$$\text{Recovery } (\%) = 2^{\text{AE} \times \left(\text{Ct}_{\text{input}} - \text{Ct}_{\text{MeDIP}} \right)} \times 100$$

Specificity of MeDIP, indexed as the ratio of methylated DNA recovery to unmethylated DNA, is calculated as:

$$\text{Specificity} = 1 - \left\{ \frac{\text{recovery}_{\text{unmeth}}}{\text{recovery}_{\text{meth}}} \right\}$$

We consider MeDIP successful when specificity is ≥ 95 % and unmethylated recovery < 1 %.

28. Purified PCR products can be stored at -20 °C for up to 3 months and longer at -80 °C

29. Multiple samples can be run on a single gel. However, maintain a minimum of 2 cm (three wells) between ladder and sample wells.

30. We excise and purify 300–350 bp libraries, which correspond to 180–230 bp insert sizes. We also excise 250–300 bp and 350–400 bp "contingency" libraries.

31. To prevent cross contamination of libraries, use a fresh scalpel for each library.

32. Because UV exposure can be carcinogenic, wear protective clothing and UV-resistant face shield.

33. The aim of QC 2 is to verify the library insert remains enriched for methylated fragments and depleted for unmethylated fragments following amPCR and gel excision. In contrast to QC 1, QC 2 involves the qPCR of fragments from just the sample DNA. This is because the λ-DNA fragments are not ligated to adapter sequences and evade amplification during amPCR. Calculate the fold-enrichment ratio for methylated vs. unmethylated regions:

$$\text{Fold Enrichment Ratio} = 2 \times \text{AE}^{\left(\text{Ct}_{\text{MeDIP\_unmeth}} - \text{Ct}_{\text{MeDIP\_meth}} \right)}$$

We recommend sequencing libraries if the fold-enrichment ratio exceeds 25, that is, the methylated fragments tested are

25-fold more enriched than the unmethylated fragments; we routinely see, however, fold-enrichment ratios greater than 100 and higher scores are better.

34. Prior to alignment, BWA should be used to index the reference genome using "bwa index", using fasta files as input (the genomic fasta files are available from numerous public repositories including the UCSC Genome Browser (http://genome.ucsc.edu/))

35. Other alignment tools such as Bowtie [14] and Novoalign (Novocraft Technologies) may also be used

Acknowledgements

The authors wish to acknowledge funding support from IMI-JU OncoTrack (115234), EU-FP7 BLUEPRINT (282510), and a Royal Society Wolfson Research Merit Award (WM100023).

References

1. Goll MG, Bestor TH (2005) Eukaryotic cytosine methyltransferases. Annu Rev Biochem 74:481–514

2. Ehrlich M, Lacey M (2013) DNA methylation and differentiation: silencing, upregulation and modulation of gene expression. Epigenomics 5:553–568

3. Lister R, Pelizzola M, Dowen RH, Hawkins RD, Hon G, Tonti-Filippini J, Nery JR, Lee L, Ye Z, Ngo QM et al (2009) Human DNA methylomes at base resolution show widespread epigenomic differences. Nature 462:315–322

4. Li Y, Zhu J, Tian G, Li N, Li Q, Ye M, Zheng H, Yu J, Wu H, Sun J et al (2010) The DNA methylome of human peripheral blood mononuclear cells. PLoS Biol 8, e1000533

5. Lister R, Pelizzola M, Kida YS, Hawkins RD, Nery JR, Hon G, Antosiewicz-Bourget J, O'Malley R, Castanon R, Klugman S et al (2011) Hotspots of aberrant epigenomic reprogramming in human induced pluripotent stem cells. Nature 471:68–73

6. Bock C (2012) Analysing and interpreting DNA methylation data. Nat Rev Genet 13:705–719

7. Down TA, Rakyan VK, Turner DJ, Flicek P, Li H, Kulesha E, Graf S, Johnson N, Herrero J, Tomazou EM et al (2008) A Bayesian deconvolution strategy for immunoprecipitation-based DNA methylome analysis. Nat Biotechnol 26:779–785

8. Beck S (2010) Taking the measure of the methylome. Nat Biotechnol 28:1026–1028

9. Eckhardt F, Lewin J, Cortese R, Rakyan VK, Attwood J, Burger M, Burton J, Cox TV, Davies R, Down TA et al (2006) DNA methylation profiling of human chromosomes 6, 20 and 22. Nat Genet 38:1378–1385

10. Pettersson E, Lundeberg J, Ahmadian A (2009) Generations of sequencing technologies. Genomics 93:105–111

11. Taiwo O, Wilson GA, Morris T, Seisenberger S, Reik W, Pearce D, Beck S, Butcher LM (2012) Methylome analysis using MeDIP-seq with low DNA concentrations. Nat Protoc 7:617–636

12. Wilson GA, Dhami P, Feber A, Cortazar D, Suzuki Y, Schulz R, Schar P, Beck S (2012) Resources for methylome analysis suitable for gene knockout studies of potential epigenome modifiers. Gigascience 1:3

13. Rakyan VK, Down TA, Thorne NP, Flicek P, Kulesha E, Graf S, Tomazou EM, Backdahl L, Johnson N, Herberth M et al (2008) An integrated resource for genome-wide identification and analysis of human tissue-specific differentially methylated regions (tDMRs). Genome Res 18:1518–1529

14. Langmead B, Trapnell C, Pop M, Salzberg SL (2009) Ultrafast and memory-efficient alignment of short DNA sequences to the human genome. Genome Biol 10:R25

Methods in Molecular Biology (2017) 1589: 139–159
DOI 10.1007/7651_2015_260
© Springer Science+Business Media New York 2015
Published online: 03 July 2016

Bisulfite Conversion of DNA from Tissues, Cell Lines, Buffy Coat, FFPE Tissues, Microdissected Cells, Swabs, Sputum, Aspirates, Lavages, Effusions, Plasma, Serum, and Urine

Maria Jung, Barbara Uhl, Glen Kristiansen, and Dimo Dietrich

Abstract

Locus-specific analyses of DNA methylation patterns usually require a bisulfite conversion of the DNA, where cytosines are deaminated to uracils, while methylated and hydroxymethylated cytosines remain unaffected. The specific discrimination of hydroxymethylation and methylation can be achieved by introducing an oxidation of 5-hydroxymethylcytosines to 5-formylcytosines and subsequent bisulfite-mediated deamination of 5-formylcytosines.

DNA methylation analysis of cell-free circulating DNA in liquid biopsies, i.e., blood samples (serum and plasma), urine, aspirates, bronchial lavages, pleural effusions, and ascites, is of great interest in clinical research. However, due to the generally low concentration of circulating cell-free DNA in body fluids, high volumes need to be analyzed. A reduction of this volume, e.g., by means of a polymer-mediated enrichment, is required in order to facilitate the bisulfite conversion. Further, these sample types usually contain a cellular fraction which is of additional interest and requires specific protocols for the sample preparation.

Formalin-fixed, paraffin-embedded (FFPE) tissue is the most commonly used source for tissue-based clinical research. Due to degradation and covalent modifications of DNA in FFPE tissue samples, optimized protocols for the DNA preparation and bisulfite conversion are required.

This chapter describes methods and protocols for the sample preparation and subsequent high-speed bisulfite conversion and DNA clean-up for several types of relevant samples, i.e., serum, plasma, urine, buffy coat, aspirates, sputum, lavages, effusions, ascites, swabs, fresh tissues, cell lines, FFPE tissues, and laser microdissected cells.

Additionally, two real-time PCR assays for DNA quantification and quality control are described. The cytosine-free fragment (CFF) assay allows for the simultaneous quantification of bisulfite converted and total DNA and thus the determination of bisulfite conversion efficiency. The *Mer9* real-time PCR assay amplifies the bisulfite converted sequence of the repetitive element *Mer9* and enables the accurate quantification of minute DNA amounts, as present in microdissected cells and body fluids.

Keywords: DNA methylation, DNA hydroxymethylation, Bisulfite conversion, Body fluids, Plasma, Serum, FFPE tissue, Effusions, Polymer-mediated enrichment, DNA quantification

1 Introduction

DNA methylation and DNA hydroxymethylation are epigenetic mechanisms, which play an important role in biological processes, such as differentiation, gene regulation, maintenance of genomic stability, epigenetic reprogramming, and pluripotency (for review: [1]). Furthermore, DNA methylation and hydroxymethylation are involved in carcinogenesis and tumor progression (for review: [2]), thereby presenting valuable biomarker candidates.

DNA methylation analyses are based on the determination of the abundance of methylated, in contrast to unmethylated, cytosines. However, methylated cytosine and unmethylated cytosine are difficult to distinguish from each other by means of conventional molecular biological techniques since they exhibit the same base pairing behavior. Frommer et al. [3] developed a protocol allowing for a deamination of cytosines to uracils while leaving the methylated cytosines unaffected. This bisulfite-mediated reaction transforms the epigenetic information into sequence information, which can be studied via PCR and other hybridization-based methods. Several technological developments have now led to improved protocols which are more convenient and user-friendly as compared to the original protocol [4–9]. The bisulfite conversion of DNA is a chemical reaction under harsh conditions. Optimal reaction conditions are characterized by low pH, high temperature, and elongated incubation times, resulting in significant DNA degradation [10–12]. Bisulfite (HSO_3^-) reacts with cytosines through the formation of a 5,6-dihydrocytosine-6-sulfonate intermediate. This reaction would preferably take place in a single-stranded DNA molecule at an acidic pH of around 5. Covalent addition of bisulfite to cytosine induces the hydrolytic deamination of the resulting 5,6-dihydrocytosine-6-sulfonate intermediate [13, 14]. Finally, bisulfite is eliminated at alkaline pH [13]. Optimal reaction conditions lead to a balance of the desired (deamination of cytosines) and undesired reactions (DNA degradation and deamination of methylcytosines). High bisulfite concentrations and high temperature at prolonged incubation times lead to a complete conversion of all cytosines to uracils but cause DNA degradation and inappropriate conversion of methylcytosines to thymines [15, 16]. An incomplete conversion of cytosines and a high rate of inappropriate conversion of methylcytosines cause false positive and false negative methylation signals, respectively, in downstream analyses [15, 16]. The main cause for DNA degradation is depurination and depyrimidation leading to abasic sites [10, 12]. These abasic sites lead to *N*-glycoside bond cleavage and therefore DNA strand breaks. High-molarity, high-temperature protocols are published which allow for a rapid bisulfite conversion within less than 1 h [7–9, 13]. These preferred conditions yield greater homogeneity of bisulfite conversion and less DNA degradation [15, 16]. Subsequent to the bisulfite reaction, a highly efficient clean-up of the converted DNA is mandatory in order to allow downstream analyses of the eluted DNA without any impairment, i.e., PCR inhibition.

In order to perform clinically relevant research on DNA methylation and hydroxymethylation, one must be able to analyze clinically relevant specimens, each of which represents specific challenges regarding the sample preparation. Furthermore, in order to reduce costs, save time, and prevent a loss of valuable sample material, a DNA extraction prior to the bisulfite conversion should be avoided.

Formalin-fixed, paraffin-embedded (FFPE) tissue is the most commonly used source for tissue-based molecular biological testing. FFPE tissue samples are widely available and inexpensive in long-term storage. In many instances FFPE tissue samples are the only available materials for retrospective clinical studies. In the clinical laboratory routine of pathologies, almost all biopsies and surgical specimens are fixed with formalin and subsequently paraffin-embedded. Accordingly, FFPE tissue samples do not only represent a valuable source for retrospective studies but are also the most important material for standard routine diagnostics. In the meantime, several methylation biomarkers in FFPE tissue samples are already in clinical use for diagnostic, predictive, and screening purposes. Methylation of *MGMT*, *PITX2*, *APC*, *GSTP1*, and *RASSF1* are in use as predictive, prognostic, and diagnostic biomarkers in glioma and prostate cancer patients [17–23]. However, DNA isolated from FFPE tissue samples is severely degraded. This fragmented DNA represents a poor substrate for molecular biological methods, e.g., PCR [24–26]. Furthermore, fixation with formalin leads to the formation of DNA–DNA and DNA–protein crosslinks, which are not completely removed by common lysis protocols [27]. Accordingly, optimized protocols for the preparation of bisulfite DNA from FFPE tissue samples are urgently needed. Additional challenges appear when analyzing minute amounts of FFPE tissues, i.e., small biopsy samples or laser capture microdissected samples.

Body fluids, i.e., blood plasma, blood serum, urine, pleural effusion, ascites, aspirates, and lavages are clinically relevant and promising sample types. In particular, blood plasma and blood serum hold the potential to improve the management of malignant diseases in the future. Tumor-specific methylation of cell-free circulating DNA in plasma has already been established as a biomarker for early cancer detection (screening), diagnostics, and prognostics [28–31]. However, methylation analysis in body fluids is challenging due to the low abundance of circulating cell-free DNA necessitating high volumes of body fluids for analyses. Accordingly, a volume reduction of the body fluid and an enrichment of the DNA are required prior to the bisulfite conversion. Furthermore, body fluids usually contain a cellular fraction (buffy coat, urine sediment, etc.) which is of interest for researchers as well. The preparation of bisulfite DNA from these samples requires protocols which are optimized with regard to the specific properties of each sample. Sputum and bronchial lavage samples for example contain mucous which needs to be degraded prior to the cell lysis.

Several published protocols and commercial kits are available giving even inexperienced researchers access to methylation analyses. However, these protocols and kits are mainly developed to enable the bisulfite conversion of extracted high molecular DNA. Only a few kits allow for the modification of DNA from challenging input sample material. The innuCONVERT Bisulfite Body Fluids Kit (Analytik Jena, Germany) is designed for methylation analyses of cell-free circulating DNA from large sample volumes up to 3 ml of body fluids. The kit has been validated for the application of pleural effusions, ascites, urine, blood plasma, and blood serum [15]. DNA from body fluids is enriched using a polymer-mediated enrichment technology (PME, Section 3.1) during which the body fluid is captured within a matrix formed by polymers. Finally, the DNA containing matrix is pelleted and dissolved in a low volume which is applicable to the subsequent bisulfite conversion and DNA purification. A second kit, the innuCONVERT Bisulfite All-In-One Kit (Analytik Jena, Germany), enables the preparation of bisulfite DNA from various cellular sample types, i.e., FFPE tissue samples, fresh tissues, and cell pellets from various sources. The protocol allows for the efficient and quick preparation of highly pure and integer DNA as needed for downstream analyses. A high purity of the bisulfite converted DNA is mandatory since the low concentration of DNA as present in several clinical samples usually requires a high volume of the eluted DNA for input into the PCR reaction. Therefore, the risk of carrying over impurities is increased. These impurities, i.e., bisulfite, wash buffers, and ethanol, might otherwise lead to severe PCR inhibition. Several very specific reagents, i.e., polymers, silica membrane spin columns, and specific bisulfite solutions, which are nonstandard laboratory reagents, are needed for an efficient and successful bisulfite conversion and subsequent DNA purification. Together these two kits provide solutions for virtually all existing sample types of clinical relevance. Due to the complexity of the bisulfite reaction, the prior enrichment and the subsequent purification, even experienced researchers usually prefer the usage of kit solutions. The protocols described in this chapter are variants of protocols contained in the above mentioned kits. These modified protocols allow for the highly efficient preparation of bisulfite DNA from challenging samples without previous DNA extraction. Protocols for plasma, serum, urine, ascites, pleural effusions, lavages, sputum, cellular fractions thereof (urine sediment, buffy coat), FFPE tissue samples (sections, punch biopsy cores, laser microdissected samples), fresh tissues, swabs, and cell lines are introduced.

Finally, quantification and quality control of total and bisulfite converted DNA can be achieved by UV spectrophotometry (Section 3.11) and quantitative real-time PCR (qPCR). The choice of a suitable qPCR assay is not trivial. One problem is the availability of standard DNA for the preparation of a standard curve. Usually, bisulfite converted DNA is used as standard DNA which suffers from degradation due to the bisulfite conversion and potentially from insufficient bisulfite conversion due to handling errors during its preparation. Two qPCR assays are introduced in this chapter. The *Mer9* assay amplifies the bisulfite converted sequence of a long terminal repeat (LTR) (Section 3.13). Multiple copies of this LTR are evenly distributed over the genome. Since bisulfite DNA is highly fragmented, this assay enables the quantification of samples which contain less than one copy of the human genome. Several sample types, e.g., body fluids and microdissected cells, usually only contain minute amounts of DNA and the whole DNA sample should be applied to the subsequent biological or clinical analysis. Accordingly, no leftover sample is available which can be used to determine the DNA quantity in a given sample. Hence, only a minor fraction of the valuable sample needs to be analyzed for quality control purposes. The CFF assay targets a locus which does not contain cytosines (cytosine-free fragment, CFF). Since the target locus does not contain cytosines within the sense strand, this strand is not altered during bisulfite conversion and therefore can be used to quantify genomic DNA as well as bisulfite converted DNA without the introduction of a bias [15]. This assay is duplexed with a second PCR targeting a bisulfite converted region within the *ACTB* gene locus (Section 3.12). This assay allows for the quantification of the total yield of DNA (including residual unconverted DNA) and the portion of converted DNA. Therefore, this assay allows for an estimation of the bisulfite conversion efficiency.

2   Materials

2.1   Sample Preparation: Cell-Free Circulating DNA

1. SB3 tube rotator model with variable speed (Bibby Scientific Limited, Stone, Staffordshire, UK # 445-2102) or equivalent.

2. innuCONVERT Bisulfite Body Fluids Kit (Analytik Jena, Germany # 845-IC-3000040): Enrichment Reagent VCR-1 and -2, Lysis Solution GS, Carrier RNA, Proteinase K, Binding Solution VL, Spin Filter, Receiver Tubes (collection tubes), Washing Solution C, Washing Solution BS.

3. Prepare aqueous proteinase K (20 mg/ml) solution.

4. Prepare carrier RNA solution (200 ng/μl polyadenylic acid).

5. Prepare the washing working solution by mixing nine parts absolute ethanol with one part washing solution BS. 1.3 ml washing working solution is required for each sample.

2.2   Sample Preparation: Cellular Samples

1. Prepare aqueous 1,4-Dithiothreitol (DTT) (0.5 g/l) solution.

2. Prepare aqueous proteinase K (20 mg/ml) solution.

3. Prepare carrier RNA solution (200 ng/μl polyadenylic acid).

4. (R)-(+)-Limonene (Merck Millipore, Billerica, MA, USA # 818407) or equivalent.

5. Histopaque-1077 (Sigma-Aldrich, St. Louis, MO, USA # 10771-100ML) or equivalent.

6. innuCONVERT Bisulfite All-In-One Kit (Analytik Jena, Germany # 845-IC-2000040): Lysis Buffer, Proteinase K.

7. innuSPEED Lysis Tube P (Analytik Jena, Germany # 845-CS-1020100) or equivalent.

8. SpeedMill PLUS (Analytik Jena, Germany # 845-00007-3) or equivalent.

2.3 High-Speed Bisulfite Conversion

1. innuCONVERT Bisulfite All-In-One or Body Fluids Kit (Analytik Jena, Germany # 845-IC-2000040 or 845-IC-3000040): Conversion Reagent, Conversion Buffer, Binding Buffer, Washing Solution, Desulfonation Buffer, Elution Buffer, Silica Membrane Spin Column.

2. Prepare the binding buffer working solution by mixing one part absolute ethanol with one part binding solution GS.

3. Prepare the desulfonation buffer working solution by mixing three parts absolute ethanol with one part desulfonation buffer.

4. Prepare the washing buffer working solution by mixing nine parts absolute ethanol with one part washing solution BS.

2.4 DNA Quantification and Quality Control

1. *ACTB* forward primer (sequence: 5′-cccttaaaaattacaaaaaccacaa-3′) (biomers.net GmbH, Ulm, Germany) or equivalent.

2. *ACTB* reverse primer (sequence: 5′-ggaggaggtttagtaagtttttg-3′) (biomers.net GmbH, Ulm, Germany) or equivalent.

3. *ACTB* probe (sequence: 5′-HEX-accaccacccaacacacaataacaaa-caca-TAMRA-3′) (biomers.net GmbH, Ulm, Germany) or equivalent.

4. CFF forward primer (sequence: 5′-taagagtaataatggatggatgatg-3′) (biomers.net GmbH, Ulm, Germany) or equivalent.

5. CFF reverse primer (sequence: 5′-cctcccatctcccttcc-3′) (biomers.net GmbH, Ulm, Germany) or equivalent.

6. CFF probe (sequence: 5′-6-FAM-atggatgaagaaagaaaggatgagt-BHQ-1-3′) (biomers.net GmbH, Ulm, Germany) or equivalent.

7. *Mer9* forward primer (sequence: 5′-ggtttttatagtttttagagttga-3′) (biomers.net GmbH, Ulm, Germany) or equivalent.

8. *Mer9* reverse primer (sequence: 5′-catcccttcttttcccat-3′) (biomers.net GmbH, Ulm, Germany) or equivalent.

9. *Mer9* probe (sequence: 5′-6-FAM-aatactaataactaacttactattaat-Dabcyl-3′) (Exiqon, Vedbaek, Denmark) or equivalent. The detection probe contains modified cytidines (LNA).

10. FastStart Taq DNA Polymerase, dNTPack (Roche Applied Science, Penzberg, Germany # 04738314001) or equivalent.

11. 7500 Fast Real-Time PCR System (Life Technologies, Carlsbad, CA, USA # 4351106) or equivalent.

3 Methods

3.1 Sample Preparation: Circulating Cell-Free DNA from Plasma, Serum, Urine, Pleural Effusions, Bronchial Aspirates

Ascites, pleural effusion, and bronchial aspirate samples can be used fixed (with formalin or Saccomanno's fixative) or naïve (*see* **Note 1**).

The DNA enrichment of high volume samples can be achieved by polymer-mediated enrichment (PME).

1. Preparation of plasma and serum (*see* **Note 2**): Separate the cellular fraction of blood from plasma or serum by centrifugation at 1,500 $\times$ g for 12 min. Transfer the supernatant into a new 15 ml centrifugation tube. Avoid carry-over of any cellular components. Centrifuge at 3,000 $\times$ g for 12 min. The supernatant can be stored at -20 °C (short-term storage up to 4 weeks) or at -80 °C (long-term storage).

   Note: Buffy coat can be prepared from the cruor as described in Section 3.4.

2. Ascites, pleural effusions, urine: Separate the cellular fraction of the body fluid by centrifugation at 4,000 $\times$ g for 10 min. Transfer the supernatant into a new 50 ml centrifugation tube. The remaining cellular fraction can be prepared as described in Section 3.5. For storage information *see* **Note 3**.

3. Mix 3 ml of body fluid, 10 µl carrier RNA solution, and 100 µl enrichment reagent VCR-1 in a 15 ml centrifugation tube. Vortex thoroughly for 10 s.

4. Add 600 µl enrichment reagent VCR-2. Vortex thoroughly for 10 s.

5. Incubate for 10 min at ambient temperature. Sediment the DNA containing matrix by centrifugation (4,500 $\times$ g, 10 min). Discard the supernatant.

6. Wash the sedimented matrix by adding 5 ml water without disturbing the pellet.

7. Centrifuge at 4,500 $\times$ g for 5 min. Discard the supernatant.

8. Dissolve the pellet in 600 µl lysis solution GS. Transfer the dissolved pellet to a new 1.5 ml reaction tube.

9. Add 25 µl proteinase K solution. Vortex thoroughly for 10 s. Incubate for 15 min at 70 °C in a water bath.

10. Centrifuge for 2 min at 14,000 $\times$ g. Transfer the supernatant into a new 1.5 ml reaction tube.

11. Add 300 µl binding solution VL. Mix by pipetting up and down.

12. Add the spin filter to the collection tube and transfer 600 µl of the sample to the spin filter.

13. Centrifuge for 1 min at 11,000 × g. Discard the collection tube containing the flow-through. Place the spin filter into a new 2.0 ml collection tube.

14. Add the residual sample to the spin filter. Centrifuge for 1 min at 11,000 × g. Discard the collection tube containing the flow-through. Place the spin filter into a new 2.0 ml collection tube.

15. Add 500 µl washing solution C to the spin filter. Centrifuge for 1 min at 11,000 × g. Discard the collection tube containing the flow-through. Place the spin filter into a new 2.0 ml collection tube.

16. Add 650 µl washing working solution (containing ethanol) to the spin filter. Centrifuge for 1 min at 11,000 × g. Discard the collection tube containing the flow-through. Place the spin filter into a new 2.0 ml collection tube.

17. Repeat **step 16** once.

18. Centrifuge at 14,000 × g for 3 min to remove all traces of ethanol. Discard the 2.0 ml collection tube and place the spin filter into a new 2 ml reaction tube.

19. Incubate the spin filter with open cap at 60 °C for 10 min in a thermal mixer in order to remove remaining ethanol.

20. Add 50 µl water to the spin filter and incubate at room temperature for 2 min. Centrifuge at 11,000 × g for 1 min in order to elute the DNA. Discard the spin filter.

21. Conduct the bisulfite conversion and subsequent DNA clean-up as described in Section 3.10.

3.2 Sample Preparation: Fresh Tissues

1. Place up to 1 mg of fresh tissue and 185 µl lysis buffer BC in the lysis tube P.

2. Homogenize the sample in the SpeedMill PLUS device by performing two runs for 45 s at 50 Hz.

3. Add 15 µl proteinase K solution.

4. Incubate for 3 h at 60 °C and 800 rpm in a thermal mixer.

5. Conduct the bisulfite conversion and subsequent DNA clean-up as described in Section 3.10.

3.3 Sample Preparation: Cell Lines

1. Centrifuge up to 1×10^6 cells for 5 min at 3,000 × g and discard the supernatant.

2. Add 45 µl lysis buffer BC and 5 µl proteinase K solution.

3. Incubate for 30 min at 60 °C and 800 rpm in a thermal mixer.

4. Conduct the bisulfite conversion and subsequent DNA clean-up as described in Section 3.10.

3.4 Sample Preparation: Buffy Coat from Plasma

1. Add 3 ml of histopaque to a 15 ml centrifugation tube and warm to room temperature.

2. Centrifuge for 1 min at 1,000 × g.

3. Dilute the cruor prepared as described in Section 3.1 in an equal volume of PBS and mix by inverting five times.

4. Add the diluted cruor carefully on top of the prepared histopaque fraction.

5. Centrifuge for 30 min at 400 × g in a swinging bucket rotor and set the centrifugal brake off. The fraction containing the peripheral blood mononuclear cells (PBMCs, buffy coat) appears between the upper plasma and PBS containing layer and the sedimented phase containing erythrocytes and granulocytes.

6. Discard the plasma as completely as possible.

7. Transfer the buffy coat fraction into a new 15 ml centrifugation tube.

8. Add 10 ml PBS and mix by inverting.

9. Centrifuge for 10 min at 250 × g and discard the supernatant.

10. Wash the pellet by adding 5 ml PBS and mix by inverting.

11. Centrifuge for 10 min at 250 × g and discard the supernatant.

12. Dissolve the pellet in 1.5 ml PBS and transfer it to a 1.5 ml reaction tube.

13. Centrifuge for 10 min at 250 × g and discard the supernatant.

14. Add 45 μl lysis buffer BC and 5 μl proteinase K solution.

15. Incubate for 3 h at 60 °C and 800 rpm in a thermal mixer.

16. Conduct the bisulfite conversion and subsequent DNA clean-up as described in Section 3.10.

3.5 Sample Preparation: Cellular Fractions from Urine, Pleural Effusion, Bronchial Aspirates, Sputum

Mucous sample material has to be pretreated with DTT as described in the following section. Sample material without mucous does not require a pretreatment and DNA extraction can be started from **step 6** of the following protocol:

1. Add 20 μl DTT solution to the cellular fraction of mucous samples prepared as described in Section 3.1.

2. Adjust the sample volume to 2 ml by addition of PBS and vortex for 5 s.

3. Incubate for 30 min at room temperature and 800 rpm in a thermal mixer.

4. Centrifuge for 10 min at 4,000 × g and discard the supernatant.

5. Open the cap of the reaction tube and dry the cell pellet at 60 °C for 5 min in a thermal mixer.

6. Add 45 μl lysis buffer BC and 5 μl proteinase K solution and vortex for 5 s.

7. Incubate for 3 h at 60 °C and 800 rpm in a thermal mixer.

8. Add 10 μl proteinase K solution, disrupt the pellet with the pipette tip, and vortex for 5 s.

9. Incubate overnight at 60 °C and 800 rpm in a thermal mixer.

10. Conduct the bisulfite conversion and subsequent DNA clean-up as described in Section 3.10.

3.6 Sample Preparation: Laser Microdissected Cells

For DNA methylation analyses the section must not be stained with hematoxylin and eosin (HE) prior to laser capture microdissection (LCM). Instead optimized staining protocols, e.g., Arcturus® Paradise® FFPE Tissue LCM Staining Kit (Life Technologies, Carlsbad, CA, USA) should be used.

1. Transfer 10 to 1×10^4 cells into a 2 ml reaction tube.

2. Add 45 μl lysis buffer BC and 5 μl proteinase K solution and vortex for 5 s. Spin down briefly.

3. Incubate for 8 h at 60 °C and 800 rpm in a thermal mixer.

4. Add 10 μl proteinase K solution and disrupt the pellet with the pipette tip.

5. Incubate overnight at 60 °C and 800 rpm in a thermal mixer.

6. Inactivate the proteinase K by incubation for 20 min at 90 °C in a thermal mixer.

7. Conduct the bisulfite conversion and subsequent DNA clean-up as described in Section 3.10.

3.7 Sample Preparation: FFPE Tissue Sections

1. Transfer one section of FFPE tissue (10 μm) into a 2 ml reaction tube.

2. Add 85 μl lysis buffer BC and 15 μl proteinase K solution and vortex for 5 s. (Note: The volume of lysis buffer needs to be upscaled in case of large samples.)

3. Incubate for 3 h at 60 °C and 800 rpm in a thermal mixer.

4. Inactivate the proteinase K by incubation for 30 min at 95 °C in a thermal mixer.

5. Incubate the sample at room temperature until the paraffin becomes solid.

6. Transfer the sample into a new 2 ml tube whilst the paraffin in the tube used for the lysis step.

7. Conduct the bisulfite conversion and subsequent DNA clean-up as described in Section 3.10.

3.8 Sample Preparation: FFPE Tissue Punch Biopsies

FFPE tissue punch biopsies necessitate a deparaffinization and subsequent rehydration procedure prior to the DNA extraction.

1. Add 1 ml limonene to the biopsy (up to 10 mg).

2. Incubate for 30 min at 60 °C and 500 rpm in a thermal mixer.

3. Centrifuge for 2 min at 16,000 × g.

4. Discard the limonene.

5. Add 1 ml limonene.

6. Incubate for 30 min at 60 °C and 500 rpm in a thermal mixer.

7. Centrifuge for 2 min at 16,000 × g.

8. Discard the limonene.

9. Add 500 μl absolute ethanol, mix by inverting, and incubate for 1 min at room temperature.

10. Centrifuge for 2 min at 16,000 × g and discard the supernatant.

11. Add 500 μl ethanol 70 %, mix by inverting, and incubate for 1 min at room temperature.

12. Centrifuge for 2 min at 16,000 × g and discard the supernatant.

13. Open the cap of the reaction tube and dry the pellet at 70 °C for 10 min in a thermal mixer.

14. Add 185 μl lysis buffer BC and 15 μl proteinase K solution and vortex for 5 s.

15. Incubate for 24 h at 60 °C and 800 rpm in a thermal mixer.

16. Add 10 μl proteinase K solution and disrupt the pellet with a pipette tip.

17. Incubate for 24 h at 60 °C and 800 rpm in a thermal mixer.

18. Add 10 μl proteinase K solution and disrupt the pellet with a pipette tip.

19. Incubate for 24 h at 60 °C and 800 rpm in a thermal mixer.

20. Inactivate the proteinase K by incubation for 30 min at 95 °C in a thermal mixer.

21. Conduct the bisulfite conversion and subsequent DNA clean-up as described in Section 3.10.

3.9 Sample Preparation: Swabs

1. Prepare aqueous proteinase K (20 mg/ml) solution.

2. Remove the swab from the stick with scissors and place the swab in a 2 ml reaction tube.

3. Add 380 μl lysis buffer BC and 20 μl proteinase K solution.

4. Incubate for 30 min at 60 °C and 800 rpm in a thermal mixer.

5. Conduct the bisulfite conversion and subsequent DNA clean-up as described in Section 3.10. (Note: The volume of the lysate may be reduced by means of a vacuum concentrator prior to the bisulfite conversion.)

3.10 Bisulfite Conversion and Clean-Up

The protocol as described in the following section (previously described [32]) enables the preparation of high quality bisulfite converted DNA (99.0 % conversion efficiency and less than 1 % unspecifically converted methylcytosines) within 2 h including purification [15]. Conversion efficiency can further be increased by adapting the reaction conditions as described in **Notes 4** and **5**. These adaptations are further applicable for the deamination of 5-formylcytosine as required for 5-hydroxymethylation analyses (*see* **Note 6**).

1. Mix the following components in a 2 ml reaction tube: 50 μl raw lysate (from cellular samples) or enriched DNA (from body fluids), 70 μl conversion reagent (*see* **Note 7**), and 30 μl conversion buffer.

2. Mix properly and spin down briefly in order to remove drops from the tube caps.

3. Incubate at 85 °C for 45 min in a water bath or in a thermal mixer (*see* **Note 8**).

4. Add 700 μl binding buffer working solution (including ethanol) to the bisulfite reaction mixture. Mix thoroughly and spin down briefly in order to remove drops from the tube caps.

5. Add spin filter to collection tube and transfer the sample to the spin filter.

6. Spin at 14,000 × *g* for 3 min. Discard the collection tube with the flow-through. Place the spin filter into a new 2.0 ml collection tube.

7. Add 200 μl washing buffer working solution (including ethanol) to the membrane of the spin filter. Centrifuge for 1 min at 14,000 × *g*. Discard the collection tube with the flow-through and place the spin filter into a new 2.0 ml collection tube.

8. Add 700 μl desulfonation buffer working solution (including ethanol). Incubate for 10 min at ambient temperature. Centrifuge for 1 min at 14,000 × *g*. Discard the collection tube with the flow-through and place the spin filter into a new 2.0 ml collection tube.

9. Add 400 μl washing buffer working solution (including ethanol). Centrifuge for 1 min at 14,000 × *g*. Discard the flow-through and place the spin filter into the same 2.0 ml collection tube.

10. Add 400 μl washing buffer working solution (including ethanol). Centrifuge for 1 min at 14,000 × g. Discard the collection tube with the flow-through and place the spin filter into a new 2.0 ml collection tube.

11. Centrifuge at 14,000 × g for 3 min to remove all traces of ethanol. Discard the 2.0 ml collection tube. Place the spin filter into a 1.5 ml reaction tube.

12. Open the cap of the spin filter and dry the spin filter at 60 °C for 10 min in a thermal mixer.

13. Add 50 μl elution buffer to the spin filter. Incubate at ambient temperature for 1 min. Centrifuge for 1 min at 8,000 × g (see **Note 9**).

14. The eluted DNA is stable for up to 4 weeks at −20 °C (see **Note 10**).

3.11 DNA Quantification and Quality Control: UV

Several clinically relevant samples yield only minute amounts of nucleic acids and a quantification using UV spectrophotometry is therefore not useful. Furthermore, carrier RNA which may be introduced into the workflow in order to increase the DNA yield interferes with the UV spectrum of DNA making an accurate DNA quantification impossible. Accordingly, a qPCR assay for the quantification of the yielded bisulfite converted DNA is used (see Sections 3.12 and 3.13). However, UV spectrophotometry can be used to determine the purity of the DNA [32]. Guanidinium thiocyanate shows an absorption maximum at 230–250 nm. The absorption maximum depends on the concentration of guanidinium thiocyanate (Fig. 1a) [32]. The bisulfite conversion reagent shows a similar absorption spectrum as compared to DNA (Fig. 1b) [32]. Guanidinium thiocyanate is contained in buffers used for clean-up of bisulfite converted DNA and represents a well-suited surrogate measure for the carry-over of impurities. Bisulfite converted DNA should show a relatively high absorption at 260 nm (carrier RNA and bisulfite converted DNA) and low absorption at 230 nm (guanidinium thiocyanate) [32]. A UV spectrum of a DNA sample suited for downstream PCR analysis is shown in Fig. 1c.

3.12 DNA Quantification and Quality Control: ACTB/ CFF Duplex PCR Assay

1. Dilute 25 mg of 5(6)-Carboxy-X-rhodamine (ROX) in 1.5 ml of prewarmed DMSO (40 °C) by vortexing for 20 s and incubation at 99 °C for 4 h at 1400 rpm in a thermal mixer.

2. Remove ROX crystals by centrifugation for 10 min at 20,000 × g.

3. Transfer the supernatant to a new 2 ml reaction tube and adjust to $OD_{580 \, nm} = 1.74$.

4. Prepare the mix of oligonucleotides consisting of 0.8 μM of each *ACTB* primer, 0.5 μM *ACTB* probe, and 0.3 μM of each CFF primer and probe. Each qPCR reaction requires 5 μl mix of oligonucleotides.

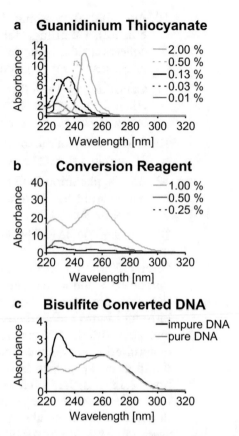

Fig. 1 UV absorption spectrum of guanidinium thiocyanate (**a**), bisulfite conversion reagent (**b**), and bisulfite converted DNA. One exemplary UV absorption spectrum from improperly and properly purified bisulfite DNA (suited for downstream PCR analysis) is shown, respectively (**c**)

5. Prepare the qPCR mastermix as follows: 70 mM Tris–HCl, pH 8.4, 12 mM $MgCl_2$, 100 mM KCl, 8 % glycerol, 0.06 % ROX solution, 0.5 mM each dNTP, and 0.2 U/μl FastStart Taq DNA polymerase. Each qPCR reaction requires 10 μl qPCR mastermix.

6. Prepare dilution series of genomic DNA and bisulfite converted DNA, e.g., 625 pg, 1.25 ng, 2.5 ng, 5 ng, 10 ng, 20 ng in 5 μl water each.

7. Transfer 5 μl of each dilution or sample in triplicate to a 96-well PCR plate.

8. Add 5 μl mix of oligonucleotides to each sample and standard DNA.

9. Add 10 μl master mix to each sample and standard DNA.

10. Perform real-time qPCR applying the following cycling program: 15 min at 95 °C followed by 40 cycles with 60 s at 56 °C,

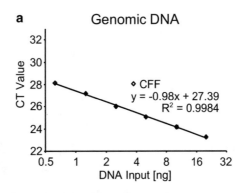

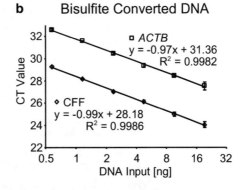

Fig. 2 Analytical performance of the *ACTB*/CFF duplex PCR assay applying a dilution series (0.625–20 ng per PCR reaction) of genomic (unconverted, (**a**)) and bisulfite converted DNA (**b**). The CFF assay amplifies a locus which is free of cytosines within the sense strand and therefore enables the simultaneous amplification of bisulfite converted and genomic DNA. The *ACTB* assay specifically amplifies a bisulfite converted target locus within the β-actin gene. Shown are mean cycle threshold values (CT values) (± standard deviation) of triplicate measurements

30 s at 70 °C, and 15 s at 95 °C. Use the following filters: HEX = *ACTB*, FAM = CFF.

11. Follow the manual of the used PCR instrument in order to calculate the concentration of total and bisulfite converted DNA in the samples. Figure 2 shows the results of the analysis of the analytical performance. It needs to be taken into account that DNA from FFPE inhibits PCR (*see* **Notes 11** and **12**).

3.13 DNA Quantification and Quality Control: Mer9 Real-Time PCR Assay

1. Prepare ROX solution according to Section 3.12.

2. Prepare the mix of oligonucleotides consisting of 0.3 μM of each *Mer9* primer and 0.2 μM *Mer9*-LNA probe.

3. Prepare the qPCR mastermix consisting of 50 mM Tris–HCl, pH 8.4, 6 mM $MgCl_2$, 10 mM KCl, 5 mM ammonium sulfate, 0.06 % ROX solution, 0.4 mM each dNTP, 0.3 μM of each *Mer9* primer, 0.2 μM *Mer9* probe, and 0.5 U/μl FastStart Taq

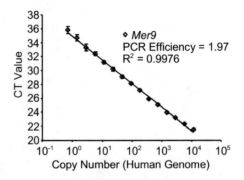

Fig. 3 Analytical performance of the *Mer9* long terminal repeat (LTR) qPCR assay applying 0.7–11,581 (2 pg–40 ng) haploid genome copies (bisulfite converted). Shown are mean cycle threshold values (CT values) (± standard deviation) of quadruplicate measurements

DNA polymerase. Each qPCR reaction requires 10 μl qPCR mastermix.

4. Prepare dilution series of bisulfite converted DNA, e.g., 20 pg, 39 pg, 78 pg, 156 pg, 313 pg, 625 pg, 1.25 ng, 2.5 ng, 5 ng, 10 ng, 20 ng in 10 μl water each.

5. Transfer 10 μl of each dilution in triplicate to a 96-well PCR plate.

6. Add 10 μl master mix to each sample.

7. Perform real-time qPCR applying the following cycling program: 10 min at 95 °C followed by 45 cycles with 45 s at 53 °C and 15 s at 95 °C. Use the following filter: FAM = *Mer9*. The analytical performance of the *Mer9* PCR assay is shown in Fig. 3.

4   Notes

1. Ethanol and other alcohols inhibit enzymes, i.e., DNA polymerases and proteinase K. A carry-over of ethanol should be avoided. Samples which are fixed using alcohol-based fixatives should be washed thoroughly using phosphate buffered saline.

2. The preparation of plasma, serum, and supernatants from other body fluids and aspirates has previously been published by Jung et al. [32]. Several systems are available for the preparation of plasma from blood. These systems differ in the way the blood is collected (aspiration or vacuum). More importantly, the collection containers contain different anticoagulants, e.g., EDTA (K2EDTA, K3EDTA), heparin, and citrate. The impact of the anticoagulant on the downstream methylation analyses is

unclear and needs to be tested carefully in each particular application. Previous studies showed that EDTA plasma is well suited for DNA methylation analyses by means of qPCR [15, 28–30]. Serum and plasma are similar regarding their preparation with the exception of the usage of the respective collection system (serum is prepared without anticoagulant). S-Monovette® (9 ml, 92 × 16 mm, Z-Gel) is a suited blood collection system for the preparation of serum for subsequent methylation analyses [15].

3. As previously discussed [32], the storability of urine samples is highly controversial. It can be observed that a storage of urine samples leads to a failing PCR amplifiability of the extracted DNA. A potential cause might be the formation of inhibitory substances during the degradation process of urine. Thus, it is recommended to prepare DNA from urine samples immediately without further storage of the urine. The prepared DNA can be stored at −20 °C.

4. A degradation of the bisulfite (see **Note 7**), improper mixing of the bisulfite reaction mixture, and an incubation temperature which is too low can lead to incomplete conversion of cytosines. Appropriate precautions should be undertaken to avoid incomplete conversion. Firstly, the temperature of the thermal mixer should be checked thoroughly. Some instruments do not work within specifications, in particular older instruments. The use of a temperature-controlled water bath is preferred to a thermal mixer. Secondly, a proper mixing of the reaction mixture is mandatory to avoid partially low bisulfite concentrations due to concentration gradients. Bisulfite is a high molar solution which tends to form two phases when an aqueous solution, i.e., DNA solution, is added. In addition, drops from the tube caps should be removed by centrifugation in order to ensure that the complete reaction volume reaches the desired temperature (85 °C). Furthermore, simple adaptations of the reaction conditions, as described in **Note 5**, can increase the conversion efficiency.

5. In order to increase the bisulfite conversion efficiency and, furthermore, to allow for the deamination of 5-formylcytosines, the following actions can be undertaken. The bisulfite concentration in the reaction mixture can be increased by adapting the composition as follows: 100 μl conversion reagent, 40 μl DNA, 30 μl conversion buffer. Furthermore, the incubation temperature can be increased to 95 °C and/or the incubation time can be prolonged to 90 min. It should be considered that these adaptations also lead to an increase in undesired conversion of methylcytosine to thymine.

156   Maria Jung et al.

6. A specific analysis of 5-hydroxymethylcytosines requires a prior oxidation of 5-hydroxymethylcytosines leading to 5-formylcytosines. The newly formed 5-formylcytosine is subsequently converted to uracil using bisulfite. This allows for the discrimination of 5-hydroxymethylcytosines and 5-methylcytosines [33]. The oxidation of 5-hydroxymethylcytosines to 5-formylcytosines is performed by means of potassium perruthenate [34]. When analyzing circulating cell-free DNA, this oxidation step can be incorporated between the bisulfite conversion step and the preceding polymer-mediated DNA enrichment (as previously described [32]). DNA from raw lysates from cellular samples should be extracted prior to the oxidation step. The TrueMethyl™ kit (Cambridge Epigenetix, CEGX, Babraham, UK) is designed to enable the oxidization of 5-hydroxymethylcytosines to 5-formylcytosines. However, deamination of 5-formylcytosine is slower in comparison to the deamination of cytosine. Therefore, harsher reaction conditions are required. Adaptations of the bisulfite reaction as described above (*see* **Note 5**) are a useful means to optimize the reaction regarding the analysis of 5-hydroxymethylcytosines (as previously described [32]).

7. The bisulfite conversion reagent contains bisulfite (aka hydrogen sulfite, HSO_3^-) and sulfite (SO_3^{2-}) [32]. Bisulfite solution liberates sulfur dioxide gas under acidic conditions. Thus the bisulfite concentration decreases over time [32]. In addition, sulfite and bisulfite are reducing agents and exposure to oxygen in the air leads to a slow oxidation of the solution to sulfate and sulfuric acid [32]. The oxidation of the bisulfite conversion reagent is indicated by a decreasing pH, lightly lucid yellow color, ammonia odor, and a decreasing viscosity [32]. When the oxidation of bisulfite reaches a critical level, the bisulfite conversion of DNA is impaired because of the low bisulfite concentration and the low pH [32]. Furthermore, sulfate might act as a potent PCR inhibitor [32]. Storage of bisulfite in the absence of oxygen is mandatory in order to increase its stability. Bisulfite solutions should not be used once expired. Bisulfite solution that is provided in single-use gas-tight vials without any oxygen is preferred. The bisulfite conversion reagent as contained in the innuCONVERT Bisulfite Kits (Analytik Jena, Germany) is stored in gas-tight vials for single use only. The bisulfite conversion reagent should not be used for more than one month once the vials have been opened. Prior to use, the pH value of the bisulfite conversion reagent should be tested using pH-paper. The performance of the conversion reagent is impaired if pH is lower than 5.1 [32].

8. The purification of the bisulfite converted DNA should be performed immediately after the bisulfite conversion reaction

in order to avoid DNA degradation. An overnight storage even at low temperatures leads to significant DNA degradation.

9. In order to yield a high concentration of the bisulfite converted DNA, the DNA should be eluted using small volumes of elution buffer. This enables the input of high amounts of DNA into the PCR at a low volume, thereby limiting the risk of carry-over of impurities into the PCR. This is of particular importance when analyzing body fluids containing a low DNA concentration (plasma, serum, and urine) and laser microdissected cells from FFPE tissues. An appropriate design of the spin column (small silica membrane) facilitates the elution using low volumes.

10. Despite other reports bisulfite converted DNA is stable and can be stored at −20 °C [15]. However, for long-term storage the bisulfite converted DNA should be buffered in 10 mM Tris–HCl, 10 ng/μl polyA, pH 8.4 [32].

11. FFPE tissues suffer from degradation of nucleic acids due to the fixation process. This degradation hampers its use significantly, impairing PCR robustness or necessitating short amplicons. However, a previous study showed that poor PCR amplification was partly caused by competitive inhibition of the DNA polymerase by fragmented DNA from FFPE tissue [26]. The optimal input of FFPE tissue DNA into PCR is 50–100 ng (according to UV quantification). Higher input amounts lead to severe PCR inhibition. This PCR inhibition can be minimized by increasing the polymerase concentration, dNTP concentration, and PCR elongation time [26]. Thus, a robust amplification of larger amplicons using template DNA from FFPE tissues can be achieved [26]. Furthermore, DNA–DNA and DNA–protein crosslinks caused by a reaction with formalin can be reverted under alkaline conditions and at elevated temperatures. Accordingly, the choice of a suited lysis buffer is highly important to yield DNA of high quality from FFPE tissues. The lysis buffer contained in the innuCONVERT All-In-One Bisulfite Kit (Analytik Jena, Jena, Germany) is optimized to allow for a complete lysis and removal of crosslinks. A prolonged lysis step for up to several days with additional supplementation of proteinase K helps to completely lyse FFPE tissues. A heat incubation step (20–30 min at 90–95 °C) after the lysis step will further remove all remaining crosslinks.

12. In addition to competitive inhibition of DNA polymerases by template DNA from FFPE tissues as described above (see **Note 11**), two other types of PCR inhibition may occur. Firstly, bisulfite salts and a low pH of the eluted DNA can lead to a bleaching of probe dyes, in particular cyanine dyes, e.g.,

Cy5, leading to an apparent inhibition. A low background fluorescence and a decrease of this background over time during PCR cycling are indicative of a bleaching of the dyes [32]. Secondly, impurities can lead to an inhibition of the polymerase, thereby impairing the PCR. The increase of the total PCR volume and the simultaneous decrease of the relative portion of eluted DNA volume in a PCR are a suitable means of decreasing PCR inhibition [32]. Usually, a 20 μl PCR reaction should not contain more than 10 μl eluted DNA. The maximum volume of input DNA might be dependent on the respective buffer conditions and the used polymerase. The maximum input volume of eluted DNA for a respective PCR system should be determined in an experiment with a dilution series of eluted DNA.

Competing Interests

Dimo Dietrich has been an employee and is a stockholder of Epigenomics AG, a company that aims to commercialize the DNA methylation biomarkers *SEPT9* and *SHOX2*. Dimo Dietrich is co-inventor and owns patents on methylation biomarkers and related technologies. These patents are commercially exploited by Epigenomics AG. Dimo Dietrich receives inventor's compensation from Epigenomics AG. Dimo Dietrich is a consultant for AJ Innuscreen GmbH (Berlin, Germany), a 100 % daughter company of Analytik Jena AG (Jena, Germany), and receives royalties from the sale of innuCONVERT Bisulfite Kits.

References

1. Guibert S, Weber M (2013) Functions of DNA methylation and hydroxymethylation in mammalian development. Curr Top Dev Biol 104:47–83

2. Sarkar S, Horn G, Moulton K et al (2013) Cancer development, progression, and therapy: an epigenetic overview. Int J Mol Sci 14:21087–21113

3. Frommer M, McDonald LE, Millar DS et al (1992) A genomic sequencing protocol that yields a positive display of 5-methylcytosine residues in individual DNA strands. Proc Natl Acad Sci U S A 89:1827–1831

4. Darst RP, Pardo CE, Ai L et al (2010) Bisulfite sequencing of DNA. Curr Protoc Mol Biol 15:1–17, Chapter 7:Unit 7.9.1-17

5. Millar DS, Warnecke PM, Melki JR et al (2002) Methylation sequencing from limiting DNA: embryonic, fixed, and microdissected cells. Methods 27:108–113

6. Boyd VL, Zon G (2004) Bisulfite conversion of genomic DNA for methylation analysis: protocol simplification with higher recovery applicable to limited samples and increased throughput. Anal Biochem 326:278–280

7. Hayatsu H, Negishi K, Shiraishi M (2004) Accelerated bisulfite-deamination of cytosine in the genomic sequencing procedure for DNA methylation analysis. Nucleic Acids Symp Ser (Oxf) 48:261–262

8. Hayatsu H, Shiraishi M, Negishi K (2008) Bisulfite modification for analysis of DNA methylation. Curr Protoc Nucleic Acid Chem. Chapter 6:Unit 6.10

9. Shiraishi M, Hayatsu H (2004) High-speed conversion of cytosine to uracil in bisulfite genomic sequencing analysis of DNA methylation. DNA Res 11:409–415

10. Raizis AM, Schmitt F, Jost JP (1995) A bisulfite method of 5-methylcytosine mapping that

minimizes template degradation. Anal Biochem 226:161–166

11. Grunau C, Clark SJ, Rosenthal A (2001) Bisulfite genomic sequencing: systematic investigation of critical experimental parameters. Nucleic Acids Res 29:E65–65

12. Tanaka K, Okamoto A (2007) Degradation of DNA by bisulfite treatment. Bioorg Med Chem Lett 17:1912–1915

13. Hayatsu H (2008) The bisulfite genomic sequencing used in the analysis of epigenetic states, a technique in the emerging environmental genotoxicology research. Mutat Res 659:77–82

14. Jin L, Wang W, Hu D (2013) The conversion of protonated cytosine-SO3(-) to uracil-SO3(-): insights into the novel induced hydrolytic deamination through bisulfite catalysis. Phys Chem Chem Phys 15:9034–9042

15. Holmes EE, Jung M, Meller S et al (2014) Performance evaluation of kits for bisulfite-conversion of DNA from tissues, cell lines, FFPE tissues, aspirates, lavages, effusions, plasma, serum, and urine. PLoS One 9:e93933

16. Genereux DP, Johnson WC, Burden AF et al (2008) Errors in the bisulfite conversion of DNA: modulating inappropriate- and failed-conversion frequencies. Nucleic Acids Res 36:e150

17. Esteller M, Garcia-Foncillas J, Andion E et al (2000) Inactivation of the DNA-repair gene *MGMT* and the clinical response of gliomas to alkylating agents. N Engl J Med 343:1350–1354

18. Stewart GD, Van Neste L, Delvenne P et al (2013) Clinical utility of an epigenetic assay to detect occult prostate cancer in histopathologically negative biopsies: results of the MATLOC study. J Urol 189:1110–1116

19. Bañez LL, Sun L, van Leenders GJ et al (2010) Multicenter clinical validation of *PITX2* methylation as a prostate specific antigen recurrence predictor in patients with post-radical prostatectomy prostate cancer. J Urol 184:149–156

20. Dietrich D, Hasinger O, Bañez LL et al (2013) Development and clinical validation of a real-time PCR assay for *PITX2* DNA methylation to predict prostate-specific antigen recurrence in prostate cancer patients following radical prostatectomy. J Mol Diagn 15:270–279

21. Weiss G, Cottrell S, Distler J et al (2009) DNA methylation of the *PITX2* gene promoter region is a strong independent prognostic marker of biochemical recurrence in patients

with prostate cancer after radical prostatectomy. J Urol 181:1678–1685

22. Schatz P, Dietrich D, Koenig T et al (2010) Development of a diagnostic microarray assay to assess the risk of recurrence of prostate cancer based on *PITX2* DNA methylation. J Mol Diagn 12:345–353

23. Weller M, Stupp R, Reifenberger G et al (2010) *MGMT* promoter methylation in malignant gliomas: ready for personalized medicine? Nat Rev Neurol 6:39–51

24. Blow N (2007) Tissue preparation: tissue issues. Nature 448:959–963

25. Bereczki L, Kis G, Bagdi E et al (2007) Optimization of PCR amplification for B- and T-cell clonality analysis on formalin-fixed and paraffin-embedded samples. Pathol Oncol Res 13:209–214

26. Dietrich D, Uhl B, Sailer V et al (2013) Improved PCR performance using template DNA from formalin-fixed and paraffin-embedded tissues by overcoming PCR inhibition. PLoS One 8:e77771

27. Kuykendall JR, Bogdanffy MS (1992) Efficiency of DNA-histone crosslinking induced by saturated and unsaturated aldehydes in vitro. Mutat Res 283:131–136

28. Church TR, Wandell M, Lofton-Day C et al (2014) Prospective evaluation of methylated *SEPT9* in plasma for detection of asymptomatic colorectal cancer. Gut 63:317–325

29. deVos T, Tetzner R, Model F et al (2009) Circulating methylated *SEPT9* DNA in plasma is a biomarker for colorectal cancer. Clin Chem 55:1337–1346

30. Kneip C, Schmidt B, Seegebarth A et al (2011) *SHOX2* DNA methylation is a biomarker for the diagnosis of lung cancer in plasma. J Thorac Oncol 6:1632–1638

31. Dietrich D, Jung M, Puetzer S et al (2013) Diagnostic and prognostic value of *SHOX2* and *SEPT9* DNA methylation and cytology in benign, paramalignant and malignant pleural effusions. PLoS One 8:e84225

32. Jung J, Kristiansen G, Dietrich D (2015) DNA methylation analysis of free-circulating DNA in body fluids. Methods Mol Biol. In press.

33. Booth MJ, Ost TW, Beraldi D et al (2013) Oxidative bisulfite sequencing of 5-methylcytosine and 5-hydroxymethylcytosine. Nat Protoc 8:1841–1851

34. Booth MJ, Balasubramanian S (2014) Methods for detection of nucleotide modification. US Patent 14/235,707, 26 June 2014

Methods in Molecular Biology (2017) 1589: 161–183
DOI 10.1007/7651_2015_264
© Springer Science+Business Media New York 2015
Published online: 03 November 2016

Analysis of Imprinted Gene Regulation

David A. Skaar and Randy L. Jirtle

Abstract

Genetic studies have been well established for identifying sequence variants associated with phenotypes. With the expanding field of epigenetics, and the growing understanding of epigenetic regulation of gene expression, similar studies can be undertaken to also define associations between epigenetic variation and phenotypes. Of particular interest are imprinted genes, which have parent-of-origin specific regulation and expression, and are key regulators of early development. Herein, we describe methods for examining epigenetic regulation by the two major hallmarks of imprinted genes: differentially methylated regions (DMRs), regulatory DNA sequences with allele specific methylation; and monoallelic expression, the silencing and transcription of opposite alleles in a parent-of-origin specific manner.

Keywords: Imprinted gene, Monoallelic expression, Bisulfite conversion, Differentially methylated region (DMR), Single nucleotide polymorphism (SNP)

1 Introduction

The analysis of imprinted genes within a sample set or population is applicable to many types of studies, but the primary intent of any such study is to determine dysregulation of imprinted genes. Such dysregulation would generally be looked for in connection to a disease state, much as population screening of genetic variants seeks to correlate sequence changes to particular conditions [1–4]. The second area of interest is in determining epigenetic changes affecting imprinted genes in connection to environmental exposures [5–7].

The study of imprinted genes includes identification of novel imprinted genes, verification of imprinting, and examining dysregulation of imprinting in sample sets. For all of these objectives, parent-of-origin epigenetic regulation is identified through allele specific gene expression, and chromosome specific methylation.

The true test of imprinted regulation of a gene, however, is parent-of-origin specific monoallelic expression. Ascertainment of this requires complementary DNA (cDNA) sequencing for informative (i.e., heterozygous) transcribed polymorphisms, so that it can be determined whether one or both alleles are being transcribed. Besides identifying imprinted genes, assays for monoallelic expression are used for determining cell-type specific gene imprinting, and in determining loss of imprinting (LOI, or biallelic expression) as related to a disease state or environmental exposure.

Expression analysis is done using single nucleotide polymorphisms (SNPs) present in genomic DNA (gDNA). Individuals heterozygous for a SNP are informative for imprinting analysis, and monoallelic expression is observed in mRNA as the expression of only one SNP allele; however, expression analysis has limitations. These include lack of available informative SNPs; low mRNA expression, which is often the case for imprinted genes in adult tissues; and that monoallelic expression exhibits spatial and temporal specificity, with transcripts that are imprinted during development often showing biallelic expression in adult tissues. Therefore, analysis of differentially methylated regions (DMRs), DNA regions that regulate imprinted genes, is a useful proxy for expression studies.

DMRs have both gametic and somatic origins, with parent-of-origin specific methylation established at gametogenesis, with subsequent creation of somatic marks after fertilization and implantation, proceeding from the gametic marks. Within the DMR, CpGs on one chromosome are methylated, and the same CpGs on the other chromosome are demethylated. DMRs are more consistent than monoallelic expression, showing less variability by age or cell type [8], and without the requirement for genetic polymorphisms, all samples can be analyzed. Therefore, for identifying an imprinted gene, finding a DMR is a simpler initial experiment, which can then be followed by the search for genes in *cis* with monoallelic expression.

Presented herein are methods for identifying imprinted genes, and determining aberrant expression, by both DMR methylation and expression analysis.

2   Materials

Nuclease free sterile water should be used for all solutions and reaction mixes.

2.1   Nucleic Acid Preparation

1. Razor blades or straight bladed scalpels
2. Buffer ATL (Qiagen, Inc., Valencia, CA)
3. Proteinase K (>600 mAU/ml) (Qiagen, Inc., Valencia, CA)
4. RNase A (100 mg/ml) (Qiagen, Inc., Valencia, CA)
5. Stat-60 (Tel-Test, Inc., Friendswood, TX)
6. Phenol–chloroform–isoamyl alcohol pH 8.0 (25:24:1)
7. Chloroform
8. 3 M sodium acetate (NaOAc), pH 5.5
9. Absolute ethanol
10. Isopropanol

2.2 Bisulfite Conversion	1. Epitect bisulfite conversion kit (Qiagen, Inc., Valencia, CA)
	2. 10 M and 3 M NaOH
	3. 10 mM hydroquinone/quinol (Sigma-Aldrich, St. Louis, MO)
	4. Saturated sodium metabisulfite, pH 5.0: 7.6 g $Na_2S_2O_5$ (Sigma-Aldrich, St. Louis, MO), 464 µl 10 M NaOH, water to 15 ml.
	5. Zymo-Spin I columns (Genesee Scientific, San Diego, CA)
	6. Buffer PB (Qiagen, Inc., Valencia, CA)
	7. 1× Buffer PE: 1 part 5× PE (Qiagen, Inc., Valencia, CA), 4 parts absolute ethanol
	8. Pellet Paint Co-Precipitant (EMD Millipore, Billerica, MA).
	9. 1 mM Tris–HCl, pH 8.0

2.3 PCR/Sequencing

1. 1 mM EDTA
2. Oligonucleotide primers, desalted, resuspended in water or 1 mM EDTA at 100 µM.
3. PCR polymerase. Platinum Taq (Life Technologies, Grand Island, NY), HotStar or HotStar Plus Taq (Qiagen, Inc., Valencia, CA).
4. 10 mM dNTP mix
5. 0 and 100 % methylated genomic DNA for controls (Zymo Research, Irvine, CA, Qiagen, Inc., Valencia, CA, or Life Technologies, Grand Island, NY)
6. SOPE resin (Edge Bio, Gaithersburg, MD)
7. Sephadex G-50 DNA grade (GE Healthcare Life Sciences, Pittsburgh, PA)
8. MultiScreen Column loader (45 µl wells)
9. MultiScreen HV 96-well plates, 0.45 µm pore size (EMD Millipore, Billerica, MA)
10. BigDye 3.1 sequencing master mix (Life Technologies, Grand Island, NY)

2.4 Cloning

1. TOPO TA cloning kit with vector pCR4-TOPO and chemically competent TOP10 or DH5α cells (Life Technologies, Grand Island, NY)
2. LB-ampicillin growth plates (Sigma-Aldrich, St. Louis, MO)
3. T3, T7, M13 forward, and M13 reverse primers (Integrated DNA Technologies, Coralville, IA)

2.5 Expression Analysis

1. Reverse Transcriptase—SuperScript III (Life Technologies, Grand Island, NY) or iScript (Bio-Rad Life Sciences, Hercules, CA)

2. TURBO DNase (Life Technologies, Grand Island, NY)

3. TwistAmp recombinase polymerase amplification kit (TwistDX, Ltd., Cambridge, UK)

4. TaqMan SNP genotyping assays (Life Technologies, Grand Island, NY)

5. Genotyping master mix (Life Technologies, Grand Island, NY)

6. MicroAmp Optical plates and optical plate seals (Life Technologies, Grand Island, NY)

3 Methods

3.1 Bisulfite Conversion of DNA

1. If genomic DNA (gDNA) needs to be purified from tissue or cell samples, extraction is performed by a cell lysis, protease, and extraction protocol.

2. 20–30 mg of tissue is used per extraction, and should be finely sliced/chopped with a sterile scalpel or razor blade, particularly if starting from frozen tissue (*see* **Note 1**).

3. Tissue is placed in a microcentrifuge tube, 500 μl Buffer ATL is added, and tissue is broken up by pipetting up and down through a 200 μl tip.

4. 20 μl proteinase K is added, thoroughly mixed by vortexing, and incubated overnight at 56 °C.

5. Samples are cooled to room temperature, then 5 μl of RNase A is added, vortexed and left at room temperature for 15 min.

6. Lysed samples are extracted by addition of 500 μl phenol–chloroform–isoamyl alcohol, vortexing, and centrifugation at 15,000 × *g* for 10 min at room temperature (*see* **Note 2**).

7. The upper (aqueous) phase is removed, taking care not to disrupt the interface, which will likely have cell debris present. The aqueous phase is re-extracted with phenol–chloroform–isoamyl alcohol up to two more times, until the interface is free of debris.

8. The clean aqueous phase is extracted once with 500 μl chloroform, by vortexing, centrifuging, and keeping the upper (aqueous) layer as for the prior extraction step.

9. DNA is precipitated by addition of 50 μL (1/10 volume) 3 M NaOAc, pH 5.5 and 1 ml (2 volumes) isopropanol and inverted to mix. Precipitate should appear as mixing occurs, and can be recovered by short centrifugation (15,000 × *g*, ~1 min), or captured in a 1000 μl pipettor tip with a minimal amount of liquid, moved to a new microcentrifuge tube and centrifuged (15,000 × *g*, ~1 min) (*see* **Note 3**).

10. The isopropanol mixture is removed by pipettor; complete removal is not required at this point. The pellet is washed

with 200 μl 70 % ethanol by vortexing and centrifugation (15,000 × *g*, 2 min). Remove as much of the ethanol as possible without disturbing the pellet by a pipettor (*see* **Note 4**), and air dry the pellet until it no longer appears wet.

11. Resuspend the DNA pellet by addition of 200 μl 1 mM EDTA and incubate at 42 °C (*see* **Note 5**). Concentration is determined by UV spectrophotometer, with $A_{260} = 1.0$ equivalent to 50 μg/ml DNA. The A_{260}/A_{280} ratio should be 1.6–1.8.

12. Bisulfite conversion of unmethylated cytosines can be done with a number of kits (such as the Qiagen Epitect kit), or with reagents made in the lab. The protocol for conversion without a kit is given here.

13. Reagents should be freshly prepared: 10 M NaOH, 3 M NaOH, 10 mM hydroquinone/quinol, and saturated sodium metabisulfite, pH 5.0.

14. Up to 2 μg DNA (*see* **Note 6**) is denatured in 20 μL, with 0.3 M NaOH (2 μl 3 M NaOH, DNA, and water up to 20 μl), at 37 °C for 20 min (*see* **Note 7**).

15. For deamination of unmethylated cytosines, 208 μl of saturated metabisulfite solution and 12 μl 10 mM hydroquinone are added, and mixed well by pipetting. Samples are incubated in the dark, at 55–60 °C for 8–12 h (*see* **Note 8**).

16. Samples are desalted with Zymo-Spin I columns. 500 μl buffer PB is added to each sample, mixed by vortexing, and centrifuged to recover droplets (12,000 × *g*, ~1 min). The entire mixture is pipetted to a spin column, which is placed in a microcentrifuge tube to catch eluate, and centrifuged at 12,000 × *g* for 2 min.

17. Collected eluate is discarded, and columns are placed back in the original tube. Columns are washed with 500 μl buffer PE, and centrifuged at 12,000 × *g* for 2 min. Eluate is discarded, and the wash step is repeated. After the second wash, spin columns are replaced in tubes and centrifuged at 12,000 × *g* for 1 min to collect residual wash buffer. Columns are placed in new microcentrifuge tubes, and DNA is eluted by addition of 50 μl 1 mM Tris-Cl, pH 8.0 and centrifugation at 12,000 × *g* for 1 min.

18. Eluted DNA is desulfonated by addition of 5.5 μl 3 M NaOH and incubated at 37 °C for 20 min. DNA is then precipitated by addition of 5.5 μl 3 M NaOAc, pH 5.5 and 135 μl absolute ethanol, mixing, and centrifugation at 15,000 × *g* for 10 min. The supernatant is removed, the pellet is washed with 100 μl 70 % ethanol (as described for DNA purification), dried, and resuspended in 20 μl of 1 mM EDTA.

19. Bisulfite converted DNA should be used for PCR as soon as possible (*see* **Note 9**).

3.2 Bisulfite PCR: Primer Design

1. Primers should be designed with 25–35 bases annealing to bisulfite converted target regions, with predicted annealing temperatures of at least 55 °C. Primer annealing temperatures should be within 1–2 °C of each other (*see* **Note 10**).

2. Primers are designed to the converted sequence of one chromosomal strand. In the primer designated as forward, cytosines from the genomic sequence are replaced with thymines. In the primer designated as reverse, guanines are replaced with adenines (*see* **Note 11**).

3. Ideally, no CpG sites will be in the primer target sequence, however, one or two CpG site in the 5' third of the primer sequence will not usually interfere with PCR amplification (*see* **Note 12**).

4. The predicted amplicon should be less than 600 base pairs (*see* **Note 13**).

5. Primer purification requires only desalting.

3.3 Bisulfite PCR: Primer/Amplicon Optimization

1. Synthesized primers are dissolved in 1 mM EDTA to a final concentration of 100 µM (*see* **Note 14**). Working stocks of primer pairs are made by mixing forward and reverse primers and diluting to a final concentration of 5 µM each primer (e.g., 5 µl forward primer + 5 µl reverse primer + 90 µl water).

2. Test PCR reactions are set up for optimizing reaction conditions. 20 µl reactions with $[Mg^{2+}]$ ranging from 1.5 to 2.5 mM are tested to identify conditions that produce single amplicons. Bisulfite converted control DNA, that is available in large amounts of high purity (e.g., commercially available DNA), can be used as template for optimization in order to not waste limited samples.

3. Reaction setup using supplied 10× buffer without magnesium (as for Platinum Taq) is: 2 µl 10× buffer; 0.6, 0.7, 0.8, 0.9, and 1.0 µl 50 mM $MgCl_2$; 0.4 µl primer mix (5 µM each); 0.4 µl 10 mM dNTP mix; 0.2–1.0 µl template DNA (bisulfite converted); 0.1 µl Taq polymerase; and water to 20 µl (*see* **Note 15**).

4. Reaction setup using supplied 10× buffer containing 15 mM magnesium (as for HotStarTaq HotStarTaq Plus) is: 2 µl 10× buffer; 0, 0.2, 0.4, 0.6, and 0.8 µl 25 mM $MgCl_2$; 0.4 µl primer mix (5 µM each); 0.4 µl 10 mM dNTP mix; 0.2–1.0 µl template DNA (bisulfite converted); 0.1 µl Taq polymerase; water to 20 µl.

5. Each range of conditions described will produce 1.5 mM, 1.75 mM, 2.0 mM, 2.25 mM, and 2.5 mM magnesium concentrations in the reactions.

6. PCR reactions should be run in 200 μl thin wall PCR tubes with caps, or plates with adhesive seals, in a thermocycler with a heated lid (105 °C). Standard cycling conditions are: heat activation (94 °C for 2 min for Platinum Taq, 95 °C for 15 min for HotStarTaq, 95 °C for 5 min for HotStarTaq Plus), followed by three-step cycling of 94 °C for 30 s, 60 °C for 30 s, 72 °C for 1 min, repeated 35 times, and a final extension step at 72 °C for 5 min (*see* **Note 16**).

7. Amplified products should be run on a 1.5 % agarose gel, made with 1× TBE buffer, using 1× TBE running buffer, and 100 bp ladder size standard. The gel is ethidium bromide stained, and visualized on a UV lightbox (using eye and skin protection). Conditions that produce intense single bands should then be used for further studies.

8. If no conditions produce single bands and/or only produce faint bands, further optimization is possible by altering annealing temperature. Annealing temperature can be adjusted from the standard 60 °C to a range from 5 °C below to 5 °C above the predicted annealing temperature of the primers. Several $[Mg^{2+}]$ can be tested against the temperature range, 0.25 mM below and above the determined best conditions. If a gradient thermocycler is available, multiple temperatures and $[Mg^{2+}]$ can be tested simultaneously, otherwise, each temperature must be tested separately.

3.4 Bisulfite PCR of Experimental Samples

1. Bisulfite PCR of experimental samples should be performed under the same conditions used to optimize PCR primers. Reactions can be run at 20 μl, or reduced to 10 μl by halving all volumes. Creation of a master mix (everything except DNA template) for a large number of samples reduces variability from pipetting small volumes.

2. 0.2–1.0 μl of bisulfite converted DNA can be used as template. The lowest usable volume is determined empirically. With >1000 ng of high-quality DNA available for bisulfite conversion, volumes ≤0.5 μl should be sufficient.

3. Amplification is verified by electrophoresis on 1.5 % agarose gel, as described under primer optimization.

3.5 Bisulfite PCR: Methylation Standards

1. Using control 0 and 100 % methylated genomic DNA, create a series of mixtures to use as standards. Intervals of 20 % are common (i.e., mix 0 and 100 % methylated at 1:0, 8:2, 6:4, 4:6, 2:8, and 0:1 ratios to generate 0, 20, 40, 60, 80, and 100 % methylated DNA). Smaller intervals (differences of 5–10 %) over a narrower range may be appropriate, once methylation amounts and typical variation for the region of interest are known.

2. Control mixtures are bisulfite converted (if controls are not already converted) and amplified under the same conditions established for each primer set, using 5–10 ng total DNA per reaction. Standards are processed through further steps just like the experimental samples (*see* **Note 17**).

3.6 Sequencing of Bisulfite PCR Products (Option 1 for Methylation Analysis: Qualitative/ Semi-quantitative Methylation Determination)

1. If sequencing facilities are available for PCR cleanup and sequencing, 8 μl of unpurified PCR product, and primers provided separately at 5 μM are usually sufficient.

2. In-lab cleanup of PCR product can be performed by ExoSAP-IT, or SOPE-sephadex columns. Both procedures can be done in 96-well plates, for working with large numbers of samples (*see* **Note 18**).

3. For ExoSAP-IT cleanup, 5 μl of PCR product is mixed with 2 μl of ExoSAP-IT reagent, and incubated at 37 °C for 15 min to inactivate unincorporated dNTPs and primers, followed by incubation at 80 °C for 15 min to inactivate ExoSAP-IT.

4. For column cleanup, a filter plate with Sephadex G-50 DNA grade is set up. Sephadex powder is poured onto a MultiScreen Column loader, and the excess scraped off and saved for later use. A MultiScreen HV plate is placed upside down on the loader, and loader and plate are inverted to transfer the powder to the HV plate. 300 μl of water is added to each well. For immediate use, allow a minimum of 1 h, and maximum of 2 h for the resin to swell. For future use, the plate can be sealed in a plastic bag and stored at 4 °C for 2–3 days. If stored, it must be allowed to come to room temperature before use. The prepared plate is placed on a standard 96-well microplate, and spun at $850 \times g$ for 3 min to remove excess water.

5. SOPE resin is added to the PCR product at 1/5 the product volume (i.e., 3 μl SOPE to 15 μl PCR product) and mixed by pipetting. The product with SOPE is added to the prepared Sephadex plate, which is placed on a clean 96-well PCR plate, and spun at $750 \times g$ for 2 min to collect cleaned PCR product.

6. If a sequencing service is used at this point to run sequencing reactions, the entire cleaned product (or 10 μl, whichever is less), and primers at 5 μM should be provided.

7. If dye-terminator cycle sequencing reactions are to be run by the researcher, they are done by a 1/16 reaction protocol. When starting with each amplicon, 2 sequencing reactions should be run for each PCR reaction, to generate both forward and reverse sequence. Each reaction includes: 0.5 μl BigDye 3.1 master mix, 1.5 μl 5× BigDye sequencing buffer, 1 μl primer for sequencing (the same primers used for PCR, used singly, at 3.2 pmol/μl), 20 ng cleaned PCR product (usually 1–2 μl), and water to 10 μl. Reactions are set up in PCR tubes

or plates, as described previously (Section 3.3) and incubated in a thermocycler with the program: 96 °C for 1 min, followed by 25 cycles of 96 °C for 10 s, 50 °C for 5 s, 60 °C for 2 min, ending with a 4 °C hold.

8. Sephadex plates for sequencing cleanup are prepared identically to those for PCR cleanup (**step 4**). The sephadex plate is spun as previously described at $850 \times g$ for 3 min on a 96-well microplate to remove excess water. No additions are required to the sequencing reactions, all are pipetted onto the sephadex, plus 10 μl water to each well. The filter plate is placed on a clean 96-well plate for collecting cleaned reactions, and spun at $750 \times g$ for 2 min. Cleaned products are delivered to a sequencing facility for analysis.

9. Sequencing results are interpreted by observing overlapping C and T peaks at each CpG site (Fig. 1). The outputs are semiquantitative, allowing determination of hypomethylation, hypermethylation, or intermediate methylation at each site. In Fig. 1, gDNA from different tissues and different individuals shows consistent partial methylation for DMR CpG sites. Sequencing of standards will indicate the degree of quantitation available, establishing the minimum difference in methylation that can be reliably measured by relative heights of C and T peaks. Qualitative and semi-quantitative comparisons can be made between samples, determining greater or lesser methylation amounts at each site.

3.7 Cloning of Bisulfite PCR Products (Option 2 for Methylation Analysis: Quantitative Methylation Determination, and Allele-Specific DMR Methylation Determination)

1. PCR products can be efficiently cloned using TOPO-TA cloning vector pCR4-TOPO for sequencing.

2. In a microcentrifuge tube, 1–2 μl PCR product is mixed with 1 μl salt solution (provided with vector), water to 5 μl, and 1 μl TOPO vector. The reaction mixture is incubated for 5 min at room temperature.

3. 2 μl of cloning reaction mixture is added to a thawed screw-top tube of competent cells, gently mixed (**not** by pipetting up and down), incubated on ice for 5 min, heat shocked at 42 °C for 30 s, and then placed on ice.

4. 250 μl room temperature S.O.C. medium (provided with competent cells) is added to transformed cells, tubes are tightly capped, and shaken horizontally (200 rpm) for 30 min at 37 °C.

5. 50 μl of the transformation is plated on a selective LB-ampicillin plate, which is incubated overnight at 37 °C (*see* **Note 19**).

6. 10–20 colonies are picked for amplification of cloned single amplicons. Cells can be directly added to PCR reactions to act as template without any processing for plasmid purification. PCR master mix as used to originally amplify gDNA, minus

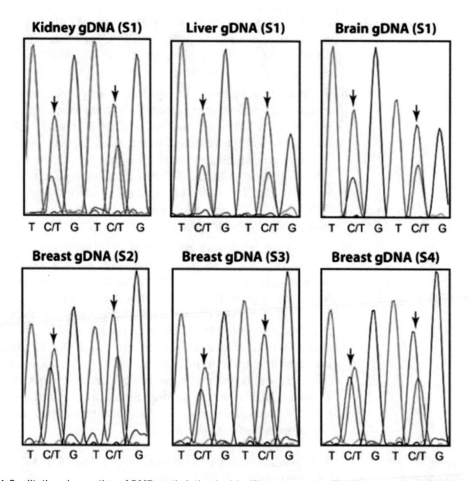

Fig. 1 Qualitative observation of DMR methylation by bisulfite sequencing. Bisulfite converted gDNA from one individual, representing each of the three germ layers (mesoderm, endoderm, and ectoderm, represented by kidney, liver, and brain, respectively), and gDNA from breast tissue from three different individuals. Neighboring CpG sites from a DMR are shown from dye terminator sequencing results. *Blue peaks* indicate cytosine (methylated CpG) and *red* indicate thymine (unmethylated CpG)

the template DNA, can be set up in reaction plates. Sterile 10 μl pipettor tips can be used to transfer single colonies to wells of the reaction plate. Soaking the tip in the mix for 1–2 min, then scraping the end against the bottom of the well before removing will transfer enough cells to the mix to amplify the plasmid. Cloned amplicons can also be amplified using primer sites in the cloning vector. T3/T7 primers or M13 Forward/Reverse primers (priming sites are incorporated into the pCR4-TOPO vector) will amplify the entire amplicon, plus flanking vector sequence.

7. Proper amplicon sizes are verified by electrophoresis on 1.5 % agarose gels, as described previously under bisulfite PCR.

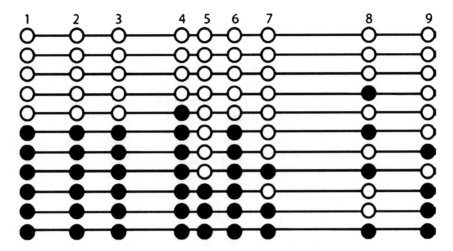

Fig. 2 Bisulfite sequencing of DMR clones. Each *horizontal line* represents one clone, *circles* represent CpG sites. *Filled circles* indicate methylated cytosines, and *hollow circles* indicate unmethylated cytosines

8. PCR reactions are cleaned and sequenced as described in Section 3.6.

9. The number of clones for which each CpG site is shown as methylated provides a methylation percentage; the more clones sequenced, the better the accuracy.

10. Sequencing of clones from the methylation standards (Section 3.5) for quantitation will show any bias in amplification of methylated or unmethylated sequence, allowing correction of experimental sample results (*see* **Note 20**).

11. For examination of allele specific DMR methylation, for each clone, the CpG sites are recorded as either unmethylated or methylated (Fig. 2). The methylation patterns across the region of interest are identified for each experimental sample, and determined to be consistent or inconsistent with allele specific methylation (i.e., the primary patterns seen are either complete methylation or demethylation of contiguous CpG sites). In Fig. 2, sites 1–3, and 6 all correlate for methylation/demethylation, indicating allele specific methylation. Site 4 also correlates to 1–3 and 6, with one exception.

3.8 RNA Preparation for Expression Analysis

1. Tissues to be used for expression analysis need to be stored to preserve mRNA. This can be done by snap-freezing in liquid nitrogen immediately upon collection, or placement in RNA-Later, followed by storage at −80 °C. Blood should be collected in PaxGene Blood RNA Tubes (Qiagen), and processed as soon as possible or frozen at −80 °C.

2. 20–30 mg of tissue will usually produce 40–120 μg total RNA, and 1–4 μg of mRNA is sufficient for multiple expression analyses.

3. Large portions of frozen tissue can be sliced with sterile scalpels or razor blades to create fragments in the 20–30 mg range. Tissue in cryotubes should be kept on dry ice, and tissue cut with a scalpel from within the tube if the tissue cannot be removed from the tube while frozen. Removal of smaller pieces of tissue can be performed by cutting on a disposable plastic weight boat (or several stacked weight boats, to prevent cutting completely through) on top of dry ice.

4. Tissue sections are sliced/chopped thinly in a weight boat on dry ice, and then immediately transferred to a microcentrifuge tube for RNA extraction.

5. RNA extraction is performed using STAT-60 (*see* **Note 21**). Approximately 10 volumes of Stat-60 are added to the tissue sample (e.g., 500 μl of STAT-60 for 20–30 mg of tissue). Disruption of tissue is accomplished by pipetting through a 200 μl tip, followed by vortexing for 30 s.

6. The tissue mixture is incubated at room temperature for 5 min, then separated into organic (lower, red) and aqueous (upper, clear) phases by addition of 0.2 ml chloroform/1 ml STAT-60. This mixture is vortexed for 15 s, then incubated at room temperature for 2–3 min, and finally centrifuged at $12,000 \times g$ for 15 min.

7. The aqueous (upper) phase is removed by pipettor with a 200 μl tip to a new microcentrifuge tube, avoiding mixing the interface between layers. RNA is precipitated from the aqueous phase by addition of 0.5 ml of isopropanol per 1 ml of the STAT-60 originally used, followed by mixing through inversion, and room temperature incubation for 5–10 min. Addition of 0.5 μl Pellet Paint co-precipitant improves precipitation and pellet visibility.

8. The RNA pellet is collected by centrifugation at $12,000 \times g$ for 10 min at 4 °C. The supernatant is removed, and 1 ml of 75 % ethanol per 1 ml of the original STAT-60 is added to the pellet. It is then washed by vortexing, and recovered by centrifugation at $7,500 \times g$ for 5 min at 4 °C.

9. The ethanol supernatant is removed, the pellet air dried briefly (5–10 min, or until no liquid is visible), and resuspended in 50–100 μl 1 mM EDTA.

10. RNA yield is quantitated spectrophotometrically, with 40 μg/ml RNA having an $A_{260} = 1.0$. The A_{260}/A_{280} ratio indicates purity, this ratio should be >1.8, ~2.0 is ideal.

11. Purified RNA should be stored at −80 °C to prevent degradation, and freeze/thaw cycles should be avoided. Aliquots of 500–1000 ng are useful for the following steps, and prevent unnecessary degradation of unused sample.

3.9 Expression Analysis of Imprinted Transcripts: Marker Selection

1. Studies of altered monoallelic expression require heterozygous DNA markers for identifying allele specific expression. Databases containing information on single nucleotide polymorphisms (SNPs) allow selection of candidate markers (*see* **Note 22**).

2. With potential markers identified, samples from the population set are genotyped to identify those informative for each SNP. Genotyping can be done by PCR and sequencing, as described above, with primers designed specifically to the SNP flanking region.

3. Rapid SNP genotyping can also be done with genotyping assays, such as probe-based TaqMan, if real-time PCR machines are available. Predesigned assays are available for most useful SNPs, and are used with genotyping master mix. The standard reaction is 10 μl, consisting of: 5 μl 2× master mix, assay probe-primer mix diluted to 1× (concentrations may be 20×, 40×, or 80×), 5 ng gDNA, and water to 10 μl.

4. Amplification reactions are performed in MicroAmp Optical 96- or 384-well reaction plates sealed with MicroAmp Optical Adhesive Film. Amplification reaction steps are: Activation of enzyme at 95 °C for 10 min, then 40 cycles of 92 °C for 15 s, 60 °C for 1 min. Completed reactions are scanned in a real-time instrument, such as the Applied Biosystems 7900HT system, identifying each individual as either homozygous or heterozygous for the SNP.

5. Multiple SNPs may be selected for a single transcript to identify more heterozygous individuals for inclusion (*see* **Note 23**), and for reproducibility of expression status on individuals with multiple informative SNPs for the same transcript.

3.10 Expression Analysis of Imprinted Transcripts: Reverse Transcription/cDNA Synthesis

1. Each marker to be reverse transcribed should have a gene specific primer (GSP) designed for cDNA synthesis. GSPs should be at least 18 bases long with predicted annealing temperatures of 55–60 °C. GSPs should be within 200–300 bases of the targeted SNP.

2. Additionally, each GSP should include a unique 5′ non-genomic tag (NGT) sequence for PCR amplification of the cDNA (*see* **Note 24**) A semi-random assortment of A, C, G, and T bases, six each, will produce a 24 base sequence with useful annealing characteristics. The semi-random criteria are: no more than two of the same base in a row, no more than six purines or pyrimidines in a row, and an A or C at the 3′ end. NGTs should be confirmed to not match genomic sequence by BLAST or BLAT searches.

3. Reverse transcription/cDNA synthesis should be performed using a polymerase with low RNase H activity, and high processivity and thermal stability, such as SuperScript III or iScript.

4. Optional treatment of RNA with DNase I can reduce background from DNA contamination (*see* **Note 25**). TURBO DNase can be used by the following protocol: nucleic acid concentration should be no more than 10 μg/50 μl, 10× DNase buffer is added to 1×, 1 μl TURBO DNase is added for up to 10 μg RNA, and incubated at 37 °C for 30 min.

5. For cDNA synthesis with SuperScript III, from 200 ng to 5 μg RNA can be used per reaction, which is set up on ice in a 200 μl PCR tube accordingly: RNA (maximum volume 6 μl), 1 μl of 2 μM GSP (or multiple GSPs, *see* **Note 26**), and 1 μl annealing buffer (provided with enzyme). Reactions are mixed and incubated in a thermocycler at 65 °C for 5 min, and then placed on ice for 1 min.

6. To the annealed RNA: primer mix, 10 μl 2× First-Strand Reaction Mix and 2 μl Enzyme Mix are added, mixed, and incubated at 50 °C for 50 min, 85 °C for 5 min, then placed on ice.

7. For cDNA synthesis with iScript, reaction setup is as follows: 4 μl 5× reaction mix (supplied), 1 μl iScript RT, up to 1 μg of total RNA, and water to a final volume of 20 μl. The reaction is incubated at 25 °C for 5 min, 42 °C for 30 min, 85 °C for 5 min and then placed on ice.

8. Control reactions include a control with no RT enzyme for detection of gDNA contamination, and a control with no RT primer, for detection of RNA–RNA priming (*see* **Note 27**).

9. Synthesized cDNA can be used in PCR reactions immediately or stored at −20 °C.

3.11 Expression Analysis of Imprinted Genes: SNP Typing in cDNA

1. Target SNPs are now PCR amplified from cDNA, using a forward primer identical to the NGT sequence of the RT primer, and a reverse primer up to 300 bp away, with the SNP(s) of interest at least 50 bases from each primer. It is ideal to place primers in separate exons if possible (*see* **Note 28**).

2. PCR reactions, cleanup, and sequencing are performed as previously described (Sections 3.3 and 3.6), using 1 μl of the RT reaction as template.

3. For low abundance transcripts, nested PCR may be required to generate sufficient amplicons for sequencing. In this case, a second pair of primers is designed, within the amplicon created by the NGT/reverse primer pair. 1/50 to 1/20 of the product of the first round of PCR is used as template for the second round of amplification with the nested primers. Other than using different primers and template, this reaction is run identically to the first.

4. Another alternative to nested PCR is recombinase polymerase amplification [9] by TwistAmp, which can amplify low abundance template in an isothermal reaction.

5. TwistAmp requires longer primers, approximately 30–35 bases, so that a forward primer can be the NGT sequence, plus part of the GSP sequence. Reverse primers are designed to the same length and positioned to produce 200–300 bp amplicons.

6. Reactions are performed in TwistAmp provided 200 µl tubes containing freeze-dried enzyme mixture, to which is added a stock made of: 2.4 µl of each primer (10 µM starting concentration), 29.5 µl of supplied rehydration buffer, template (1–2 µl), and water to a final volume of 47.5 µl. After rehydration of the enzyme, the reaction is initiated by addition of 2.5 µL MgAc (280 mM, supplied with enzyme mix) and incubated for 20–30 min at 37–39 °C.

7. Amplification of cDNA targets is confirmed by electrophoresis on 1.5 % agarose gels.

8. The results of sequencing are analyzed by observing single or overlapping base reads at the position of the SNP. Figure 3 shows a SNP from an imprinted gene, showing heterozygosity in gDNA, and monoallelic expression in breast cell cDNA from two individuals, expressing alternate bases.

9. An alternative to dye terminator sequencing is to use Taqman genotyping assays on the synthesized cDNA (*see* **Note 29**). Reactions are run as for genotyping DNA, with 1 µl of the reverse transcriptase reaction as template.

10. Output of the reaction will indicate homozygous (monoallelic) or heterozygous (biallelic) expression of the SNP for each sample (Fig. 4). Samples typed as heterozygous in gDNA (Fig. 4a, 16246 and 17432, indicated) show homozygosity when typed in cDNA, clustering with cDNA from individuals

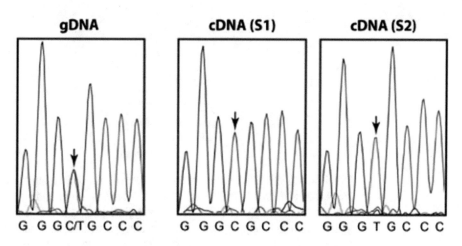

gDNA **cDNA (S1)** **cDNA (S2)**

G G GC/T G C C C   G G G C G C C   G G G T G C C C

Fig. 3 Monoallelic expression by bisulfite sequencing. A SNP from a normally imprinted gene, with C (*blue*) and T (*red*) alleles, dye-terminator sequencing of gDNA from a heterozygous individual, and cDNA from two heterozygous individuals

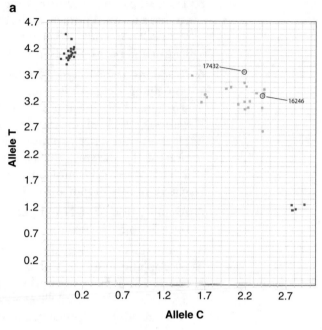

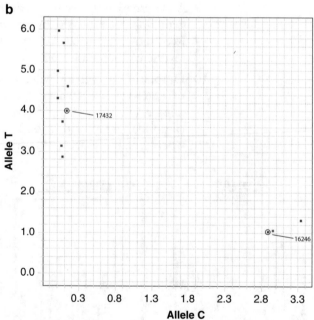

Fig. 4 Monoallelic expression analysis by TaqMan. (**a**) Genotyping of gDNA for an exonic SNP in an imprinted transcript, showing samples forming three clusters: TT homozygous (*blue*), CC homozygous (*red*), and CT heterozygous (*green*). Two heterozygous samples (indicated) were also used for typing in cDNA. (**b**) Genotyping of cDNAs from brain RNA for the same SNP. Samples repeated from gDNA heterozygous cluster are indicated

homozygous for gDNA (Fig. 4b). With biased, but not fully monoallelic, expression, the degree of biallelic expression can be determined by real time PCR comparing amplification between matching gDNA and cDNA samples. By calculating the detection threshold for each allele, the relative copy number of each can be determined, with the gDNA ratio setting a baseline for determining bias in the cDNA.

4   Notes

1. For most tissues, incubation in buffer ATL and proteinase K effectively lyses cells and digests proteins without the need for aggressive homogenization. However, particularly fibrous tissues (i.e., muscle, skin) may need mechanical homogenization.

2. Phenol and chloroform are both toxic and skin irritants, with chloroform being classified as a probable human carcinogen. Eye protection, gloves, and lab coats should be worn when working with these chemicals. The waste is treated as hazardous, and must be stored and disposed of in accordance with local hazardous waste procedures.

3. Isopropanol will initially form a layer on top of the aqueous solution; the two layers are soluble in each other upon mixing. The precipitating DNA will appear as white strings at the interface between the two solvents as mixing occurs, and will coalesce into a pellet.

4. Genomic DNA is slow to resuspend even under ideal circumstances, over-drying of the pellet increases the difficulty. One method of drying is to pour off the liquid after centrifugation (into an appropriate alcohol waste container), blot the lip of the tube on an absorbent lab wipe, and then centrifuge again to collect droplets. The droplets can be removed with a fine 10 μl pipette tip, and the pellet air-dried for only 1–2 min, or until no liquid remains visible.

5. Resuspension may require overnight incubation. It is best to start with 200 μl of 1 mM EDTA, and then determine the success after incubation. If, after 42 °C incubation, the solution is "gummy" when flicked or pipetted, more solution can be added, 100–200 μl at a time, with reincubation at 42 °C for 30–60 min, repeating as necessary until the pellet is completely in solution (do not go over 1000 μl). The pellet can absorb water and become clear, but not be dissolved. Flicking the tube and observing bubbles trapped in the pellet, or pipetting with a 200 or 1000 μl tip to find the gummy pellet will identify incomplete suspension.

6. 10–2000 ng of DNA can be bisulfite converted by kit or the method given here. Successful PCR later is dependent on the

quality of the starting DNA; bisulfite conversion fragments DNA, low quality input generates very low quality output. If low amounts of input DNA are all that is available, using a kit is highly recommended, as recovery tends to be better and kits have adapted methods for low input, including the addition of carrier RNA.

7. Complete denaturation is essential for conversion as bisulfite cannot effectively react with base-paired cytosines. If, for any reason, circular DNA is being converted (i.e., a vector insert), it must be nicked or cut with a restriction enzyme before the denaturation step.

8. Temperature cycling may improve conversion efficiency over isothermal incubation. The faster that conversion is achieved, the less damage is done to the DNA by bisulfite exposure. Periodic heating to 95 °C to re-denature DNA can allow for shorter incubation. A common protocol is: 95 °C for 5 min, 60 °C for 25 min, 95 °C for 5 min, 60 °C for 85 min, 95 °C for 5 min, 60 °C for 175 min.

9. Bisulfite converted DNA can be stored at 4 °C for up to 1 week, at −20 °C for 1–2 months, and −80 °C for 6 months.

10. A number of prediction tools are available online, that calculate not only annealing temperatures but also hairpins, and self- or hetero-dimers. http://www.idtdna.com/analyzer/Applications/OligoAnalyzer and http://www.sigmaaldrich.com/life-science/custom-oligos/custom-dna/learning-center/calculator.html (requires free registration) are two such useful tools.

11. Primer design by hand is very tricky for the inexperienced, requiring consideration of each strand separately, and proper base substitution for converted cytosines. Several useful online tools will design primers from genomic sequence without the risks of misconverting DNA, such as http://bisearch.enzim.hu and http://epidesigner.com. The epidesigner site designs primers with tags specific to the Sequenom MassArray system, which can be excluded if that system is not being used. Epidesigner can also design primers to tile across large regions, and identifies CpG sites covered by primers.

As an example, to manually design primers to this simplified dsDNA sequence:

5′ GATC......TCAG 3′ (sense)

3′ CTAG......AGTC 5′ (antisense)

Only one strand will be amplified by a primer pair after conversion, as the strands are no longer complementary:

5′ GATT......TTAG 3′ (converted sense)

3′ TTAG......AGTT 5′ (converted antisense)

"Reverse" primers are designed to anneal to the converted DNA, and "forward" primers are designed to anneal to the product of reverse primer extension (matching the converted strand, and not complementary to the converted antisense). To amplify from the sense strand of the example:

(forward primer) 5′ GATT ———>

5′ GATT......TTAG 3′

<——— AATC 5′ (reverse primer)

To amplify the antisense strand of the example, the reverse primer would begin 5′AATC, and the forward would begin 5′ TTGA. Thorough primer design can include primers to amplify both sense and antisense strands, as amplification of one may be more efficient.

A rule of thumb to quickly catch common errors is that the forward primer should have no 'C's, and the reverse primer no 'G's.

12. Deliberately including one or two CpG sites near the 5′ end of the primer is a method for reducing PCR bias that often preferentially amplifies unmethylated sequences. Primers are synthesized with only 'C' at these positions, which will allow annealing to both methylated and unmethylated DNA, but improve amplification of the methylated strand [10].

13. Verification that primers should produce an amplicon, by in silico ePCR, is a final check that no sequence mixups were made in design. Also, ePCR can identify potential unintended amplicons, as the loss of one base increases potential primer matching sites throughout the genome. This can be a particular problem with regulatory regions, which often contain similar sequence motifs. The BiSearch primer design tool (http://bisearch.enzim.hu) has an ePCR function that compares primers to in silico bisulfite converted genomes, identifying redundant primer hybridization, and all predicted amplicons from perfect and near matches of primers pairs.

14. Resuspension is aided by primer suppliers commonly reporting the primer yield in nmol. Multiply the nmol by 10, and add that many microliters of 1 mM EDTA to produce 100 μM primer stock. Some suppliers now provide this volume with primer yield data. Primers can also be resuspended in water, but EDTA is used to protect from cation contaminants, which can cause primer fragmentation. This level of EDTA will not affect further reactions, but if primers are in higher EDTA concentrations (>10 mM), this can reduce Mg^{2+} availability in PCR reactions, inhibiting amplification. Increasing Mg^{2+} in the reaction will overcome this inhibition.

15. The amount of template DNA required is variable, depending on the amount and quality of DNA input to bisulfite conversion. If at least 500 ng of DNA was used, <0.5 μl should be sufficient.

16. The extension temperature can be reduced to 66–68 °C as one attempt to improve yield, particularly with primers that have lower annealing temperatures. If reducing the extension temperature, increasing extension time by 15–30 s is suggested, to compensate for lower polymerase activity.

17. Adjustments can be made to PCR conditions to reduce bias when sequencing results for the standards are known. As mentioned in **Note 11**, primer design can reduce bias and increasing annealing temperature to the highest working temperature can also reduce preferential amplification of unmethylated DNA by reducing secondary structure in the methylated DNA [11].

18. Cleanup methods are a matter of personal preference, depending on which method is more convenient, or has produced better results for the researcher. ExoSAP-IT is a simpler protocol, but the SOPE-Sephadex method may be preferred for cost (~$0.40 per sample, compared to $0.60–2.00/sample for ExoSAP-IT, depending on scale). For purity of yield, the Sephadex columns desalt, as well as physically remove dNTPs and primers, not just inactivate them. Also, if Sephadex is being used for sequencing cleanup, the materials are already on hand.

19. The volume of cells plated can be varied depending upon the expected colony number based on experience. If plating <50 μl, the volume should be increased with S.O.C., so that it will spread evenly over the entire plate. Background with TOPO-TA vectors is low, producing a small proportion of transformants without inserts. However, the vector and cells are compatible with blue–white selection on Xgal plates, if confirmation of insert is desired before PCR. 40 μl of Xgal stock (20 mg/ml DMSO) is spread per plate, and allowed to dry before plating transformed cells. Transformants with empty vector will appear blue, those with insert containing vectors will be white.

20. After bisulfite conversion, methylated and unmethylated DNA may not amplify equally. For any quantitative work, determining this bias by sequencing a range of methylation standards is needed for validation. Standard curves can allow mathematical correction of data and determine if quantitation is most reliable over a specific range. Actual methylation results may be off by 10–20 %, and for a large actual range of methylation, a very small difference may is measured (i.e., standards from 0 to 40 % show a measured range of only 10 %). Regression of the standard curve can correct experimental measures [12].

21. Stat-60 is based on the original single-step RNA purification protocol using acid guanidinium thiocyanate–phenol–chloroform extraction [13]. Many alternatives to Stat-60 are based on eliminating phenol and chloroform and the handling difficulties they create. However, Stat-60 yields and quality are often superior to kit methods, due to the nucleic acid separation properties of acid phenol (DNA is soluble in phenol at low pH, RNA is not), highly efficient removal of proteins (including RNases) by phenol, and increased stability of RNA at acidic pH.

22. Multiple genomic databases contain SNP data, greatly simplifying the process of choosing markers. The UCSC genome browser (http://genome.ucsc.edu), The International HapMap Project (http://hapmap.ncbi.nlm.nih.gov), GenBank (https://www.ncbi.nlm.nih.gov/genbank/), and 1000 Genomes (http://www.1000genomes.org) have comprehensive lists of SNPs, including average and ethnicity specific minor allele frequencies (MAF). The most useful polymorphisms have high MAF (>0.25), are exonic and are positioned near splice sites. High MAF SNPs will allow inclusion of more samples and exonic SNPs near splice sites reduce gDNA contamination by allowing PCR to target spliced, mature mRNA. If no other options exist, intronic SNPs can be used, as they are present in pre-mRNA transcripts. However, pre-mRNAs are likely present at lower levels, making amplification difficult (nested PCR or TwistDX, as described, may be required) and will amplify identically to gDNA, making careful contamination control essential. RT primer design with NGTs can greatly improve specificity with intronic SNPs (*see* **Note 24**).

23. When selecting multiple SNPs, pay attention to linkage disequilibrium (LD) between SNPs. SNPs in high LD will have similar or identical homozygosity and heterozygosity in individuals and will not increase the number of informative samples. HapMap SNP data (http://hapmap.ncbi.nlm.nih.gov) includes LD for many SNPs, and should be used when selecting multiple markers in the same region.

24. Use of the NGT can almost completely reduce contamination from gDNA and antisense RNA, which can cause results to incorrectly appear heterozygous [14]. By using one PCR primer to target the NGT, only the transcript targeted by the RT-NGT primer sequence in cDNA synthesis is amplified.

25. PCR with NGTs can usually function cleanly in the presence of contaminating DNA, but DNase removal may still be desired; however, each additional step increases opportunities for RNA degradation.

26. More than one RT primer can be used in a single reaction, as long as the total reaction volume is not exceeded. If a particular

combination is to be used often, a master mix of RT primers can be made to keep the volume low. If using NGTs, each RT primer should have a different NGT.

27. With the findings that noncoding transcripts and miRNAs are very common, it is recognized that endogenous RNA fragments may prime antisense transcripts, which can then be amplified and obscure the results, if the antisense is not imprinted while the sense is. Avoiding this issue is a reason for using NGTs.

28. Amplification across a splice site is an effective control for gDNA contamination. If the intron is large, no gDNA PCR product will be made, and if small enough to amplify, size differences of cDNA and gDNA amplicons are visible by agarose gel electrophoresis.

29. Validated TaqMan assays have small (<150 bp) amplicons, and preset primer sequences. Their use with cDNA is not compatible with most of the RT design adaptations to avoid contamination. Removal of gDNA is therefore more critical, and even then, TaqMan assays work best with highly expressed imprinted genes. High expression in the cell type used should be confirmed, and controls for gDNA/antisense RNA contaminants run with test cDNAs for each assay, before attempting TaqMan detection in experimental samples.

References

1. Court F, Martin-Trujillo A, Romanelli V et al (2013) Genome-wide allelic methylation analysis reveals disease-specific susceptibility to multiple methylation defects in imprinting syndromes. Hum Mutat 34:595–602

2. Docherty LE, Rezwan FI, Poole RL et al (2014) Genome-wide DNA methylation analysis of patients with imprinting disorders identifies differentially methylated regions associated with novel candidate imprinted genes. J Med Genet 51:229–238

3. Horsthemke B (2014) In brief: genomic imprinting and imprinting diseases. J Pathol 232:485–487

4. Girardot M, Feil R, Lleres D (2013) Epigenetic deregulation of genomic imprinting in humans: causal mechanisms and clinical implications. Epigenomics 5:715–728

5. Rozek LS, Dolinoy DC, Sartor MA et al (2014) Epigenetics: relevance and implications for public health. Annu Rev Public Health 35:105–122

6. Murphy SK, Adigun A, Huang Z et al (2011) Gender-specific methylation differences in relation to prenatal exposure to cigarette smoke. Gene 494:36–43

7. Cooper WN, Khulan B, Owens S et al (2012) DNA methylation profiling at imprinted loci after periconceptional micronutrient supplementation in humans: results of a pilot randomized controlled trial. FASEB J 26:1782–1790

8. Murphy SK, Huang Z, Hoyo C (2012) Differentially methylated regions of imprinted genes in prenatal, perinatal and postnatal human tissues. PLoS One 7, e40924

9. Piepenburg O, Williams CH, Stemple DL et al (2006) DNA detection using recombination proteins. PLoS Biol 4, e204

10. Wojdacz TK, Hansen LL, Dobrovic A (2008) A new approach to primer design for the control of PCR bias in methylation studies. BMC Res Notes 1:54

11. Shen L, Guo Y, Chen X et al (2007) Optimizing annealing temperature overcomes bias in bisulfite PCR methylation analysis. Biotechniques 42:48–58

12. Moskalev EA, Zavgorodnij MG, Majorova SP et al (2011) Correction of PCR-bias in

quantitative DNA methylation studies by means of cubic polynomial regression. Nucleic Acids Res 39, e77

13. Chomczynski P, Sacchi N (2006) The single-step method of RNA isolation by acid guanidinium thiocyanate-phenol-chloroform

extraction: twenty-something years on. Nat Protoc 1:581–585

14. Pinto FL, Svensson H, Lindblad P (2006) Generation of non-genomic oligonucleotide tag sequences for RNA template-specific PCR. BMC Biotechnol 6:31

Methods in Molecular Biology (2017) 1589: 185–203
DOI 10.1007/7651_2015_316
© Springer Science+Business Media New York 2015
Published online: 10 April 2016

Statistical Methods for Methylation Data

Graham W. Horgan and Sok-Peng Chua

Abstract

Methylation data are continuous variables with most values in a sample lying in a narrow range. In a research project they can either be the outcome, or a variable potentially explaining some of the variation in other outcomes. A range of statistical methods are appropriate depending on the experimental questions. Before the formal analysis is carried out, it is important that data are checked and cleaned. Where batch effects may be present, this should be accounted for in the analysis. Where many methylation sites are investigated in a study, attention should be given to multiple comparisons and false discovery rates, and multivariate methods such as principal component analysis may be useful.

Keywords: Batch effects, Linear model, Regression, Statistical power, Principal component analysis

1 Introduction

Methylation values are generally percentages, so constrained to lie between 0 and 100 %. In population epigenetics the data typically consists of methylation values at one or more sites in the genome, recorded on each individual sampled. Usually there will also be other information recorded on each individual and there will be interest in the links between this information and the methylation values. The other information can be of a wide variety of types, e.g., age, gender, BMI, disease status, or lifestyle information. It may also be group membership, such as case/control, ethnicity, or treatment group.

In considering the association between methylation and other variables, we may regard the methylation values as either an outcome or an explanatory variable. They play a different role in the statistical modeling in each case and the choice may be determined by the experimental question.

2 Materials

A computer and suitable software are required for statistical analysis.

2.1 Hardware

For most purposes, any modern computer will be adequate. If very-high-dimensional methylation is collected, such as that produced by bead chip arrays, and with larger sample sizes, then high-performance computing hardware may be needed. This will be because of the greater demand for memory storage, and in order to carry out computations in a tolerable amount of time. A high-performance computer will usually consist of a number of processing units (generally termed nodes) which share the computational task either by independently working on different parts of it or by using suitable software to communicate with each other while they subdivide large computational tasks. Extra RAM (random access memory) that is used during the computation is also generally made available.

2.2 Software

There are several statistical software packages which can carry out the sort of analyses discussed below. The ones which are most widely used are (in alphabetical order):

Genstat: originally developed for agricultural research and with strong capabilities for analysis of variance and mixed modeling (www.vsni.co.uk/genstat).

Minitab: easy to use and good for data exploration (www.minitab.com).

R: open source and with a huge array of add-on libraries, it is the most widely used package among professional statisticians. It lacks a graphical user interface that can access most of its capabilities (www.r-project.org). Specific libraries of routines are available for methylation array data, such as ChAMP (http://bioconductor.org/packages/release/bioc/html/ChAMP.html) and Methylumi (http://www.bioconductor.org/packages/release/bioc/html/methylumi.html).

SAS is the main program used in the pharmaceutical industry and is much used for analyzing data from clinical trials (www.sas.com).

Stata is widely used in econometrics and also in epidemiology (www.stata.com).

SPSS has its origins in social sciences, and has been growing in popularity in many fields of biological science (www.ibm.com/software/analytics/spss/).

2.3 Other Online Resources

A variety of online resources are valuable when studying methylation data. Pathway databases such as KEGG (http://www.genome.jp/kegg/) or Pathway Commons (http://www.pathwaycommons.org/about/) can provide information on biological pathways that can be used to structure the examination of methylation at different sites. Where array data are collected, associated information about the arrays will be accessible on the manufacturer's website.

3   Methods

The approaches to studying and analyzing the data will depend on the purpose for which it was collected and the nature of the study design. A first broad division can be into experimental and observational studies and most methylation studies to date fall into the latter category. There are several common types of such studies.

3.1   Types of Study

1. *Case–control study:* This is a study in which a selection is made of subjects in which a disease or some other outcome has occurred, and another selection is made of subjects in which it has not occurred, but which are similar in other demographic respects to the case group. Any differences between these two groups in their exposure to some hazard can give us information on the extent to which the hazard influences risk of the disease or other outcome [1–3].

2. *Cross-sectional study:* This is a study which looks at a set of subjects at a single point in time, and allows us to study associations between different characteristics which are recorded on each individual. Here, we assume that methylation status is one of the characteristics recorded [4–6].

3. *Longitudinal study:* This is a study which records how subject characteristics change over time. We can then examine associations between these changes, and between the changes and the subject characteristics at the start. It is due to the nature of such studies that they take longer to conduct and to produce results. They may even last more than one lifetime in the case of transgenerational studies [7–9].

4. *Cohort study:* This is a form of longitudinal study in which a group of people are observed for a period of time in order to see which of them contract a disease or some other outcome. The factors which influence the risk of this occurring can then be studied [10, 11].

3.2   Data Management, Checking, Cleaning, Missing Values, and Batch Effects

Methylation values are often collected from samples that are handled in batches (e.g., from arrays or 96-well plates). It is possible for batch differences to arise, i.e., differences between samples in different batches that have no biological origin. This is technical variation that has a particular structure. It adds no biological information to a study and is a nuisance. Clearly it is desirable to reduce the magnitude of any batch effects, and a careful researcher will naturally try to do so. But often they cannot be eliminated completely. There are a number of ways to mitigate their effect on the interpretation of the resulting data.

1. Avoid confounding batch effects with anything of interest. Although it may be easier to manage, it is important always to avoid making batches from samples in any grouping of interest.

So sample batches should not consist of cases only and controls only, or particular treatment groups, or be analyzed in batches characterized by anything that is to be compared. If they are, the comparisons will be confused with comparisons between batches, and it will be impossible to know whether differences or associations are true biological effects or just batch differences resulting from analytical variation (*See* **Note 1**).

2. Normalization
This involves a processing step in generating the methylation values which attempts to make the measurements on each batch similar and so free of batch effects (*see* **Note 2**). There are a variety of approaches for doing this. A review in the context of bead chip assays is given in ref. [12].

3. Include reference samples
This is arguably a variation on the normalization approach, in which a particular sample is included in all batches. It should have the same methylation measurement each time, and so the differences reflect batch effects. By replacing all other methylation measurements with differences or ratios to the value of this reference sample, batch effects are theoretically removed. Although this can help to remove batch effects it will usually not do so completely. This is because a single or small number of reference samples will not capture all of a batch effect and will be subject to additional random analytical variation.

4. Include batch effects in the statistical analysis.
This is straightforward to do and should be considered even if one or more of the previous strategies are also used. To do this, create a factor in the data file to record which batch an observation was obtained from. Then include this batch term in the statistical model for analyzing the data. Variability between batches will then be accounted for by that term, and will not appear in the residual (unexplained) variability. The residual variability will therefore be reduced, which will lead to lower standard errors and more significant *p*-values (*see* **Note 3**).

3.3 Choosing an Approach to Analysis

1. Linear models
Analysis of methylation data will generally consist of constructing a statistical model of the data, to relate the methylation values to the other data collected on each subject. There will usually be several methylation values obtained for each subject, possibly very many in the case of array analysis. We may consider these one at a time, looking for patterns in the results of these analyses, or handle them jointly in a single analysis. If the number of methylation variables exceeds about ten, some of *dimension reduction* is likely to be useful. These are methods, such as principal component analysis (PCA), which aim to capture, in a small number of components, most of the

variation of interest in a larger set of variables. PCA aims to find linear combinations of the original variables, with each component uncorrelated with the others and maximizing the amount of variation that is contained in the original variables.

The routinely used statistical models are all variations of a linear model. They assume that the mean of the outcome (response) variable may be expressed as a linear combination of the other (explanatory) variables. The methylation variables may play the role of either outcome or explanatory variable. So if we denote the outcomes as Υ and the explanatory variables as X_1, X_2, X_3, etc., then the model states that

$$\Upsilon = \beta_1 X_1 + \beta_2 X_2 + \beta_3 X_3 + \cdots + \varepsilon.$$

Each β value is termed a coefficient, and indicates how changes in the corresponding X variable affect Υ, on average. The final term ε denotes random variation independent of any of the X variables. We usually also add the assumption that this random variation is normally distributed.

The above model was written on the basis of the X variables being continuous measurements. If any explanatory variates are categorical (e.g., if they specify and code group membership) then they are incorporated in the model as indicator variables. One group is arbitrarily denoted as the reference group or level, and an extra variable is created for each other group, which is 0 for all observations apart from those in the corresponding group, for which it is 1 (*see* **Note 4**).

When a model if fitted to a set of data, a number of results are obtained:

- Estimates of the values of the β coefficients

- Standard errors of these estimates

- P-values to test whether the values differ significantly from zero

- An estimate of the variance of ε

- R^2—this may be interpreted as the proportion of the variance of Υ that can be explained by the variability in X. An adjusted version, which accounts for the amount of variation that is randomly explained by ε, can be presented.

The p-values are often of primary interest, as they are a quantification of the evidence that the corresponding β is not zero, and so the explanatory variable has some association with the outcome, after adjustment for the other variables. Formally, the p-value is the probability of a β value as large as the one estimated occurring by chance in the absence of any association. So small p-values indicate evidence for an association, and the smaller the p-value the stronger the evidence. They can be seen as a common scale for evidence, which has the same interpretation whatever the scientific topic, type of data, or statistical method involved.

2. Quantiles

It is common to handle continuous variables by dividing the range of values into intervals to produce an ordered categorical variable. The main reason for doing this is convenience. It can be easier to interpret the differences between these categories than to talk about the effects of gradual changes in the continuous variable. In some cases, statistical analysis using these categories is more easily able to account for effects such as nonlinearity, which require more care on the continuous scale.

The definition of the intervals can be done in various ways. Dividing age into decade intervals (20–30, 30–40, etc.) seems natural and body mass index is traditionally divided into intervals of <18, 18–25, 25–30, and >30 as a choice of readily remembered round numbers which seem to health scientists to be a suitable division. Splitting the range of values according to the distribution is also widely done. This involves choosing dividing points so that the same proportion of observations fall into each interval. The usual choices are three intervals (tertiles) or four (quartiles) or five (quantiles) and occasionally ten (deciles). This ensures an equal number of observations in each category, which is optimal for statistical power (*see* **Note 5**).

3.4 The Normal Distribution

In most linear models, the probability calculations involved in obtaining *p*-values assume that the residual part of the variation is normally distributed. This should be checked before model fitting. If the variation due to effects of interest is small compared to the residual variation, then we can expect that the distribution of the original values will be close to normal also, and so it is common to check this before model fitting (*see* **Note 6**).

How close a distribution is to normality can be assessed by examining a histogram or a normal probability plot (a special case of what is termed a Q–Q plot). The latter plots the normal score of each data value (where on a standard normal distribution the point would be, based on its rank in the data) against the data value itself, sometimes scaled by the standard deviation and centered to zero mean. For data which do come from a normal distribution, this should be approximately a straight line.

Figure 1 shows an example of a histogram (Fig. 1a) and normal probability plot (Fig. 1b) for some methylation data. In this case, assumptions of normality seem to be reasonably justified. How important assumptions of normality are, and how robust the tests are to failure of these assumptions, has been studied, and some references are [13, 14]. Transforming data values before analysis, such as by taking logs or square roots, can make skewed distributions approximately normal, and thereby ensure that statistical tests based on them are more reliable (*see* **Note 7**). Nonparametric tests

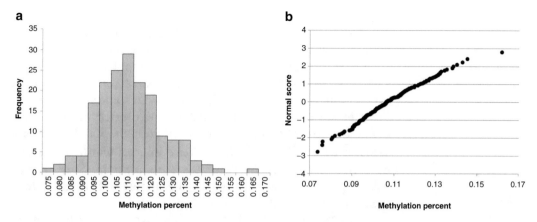

Fig. 1 (**a**) Histogram and (**b**) normal score plot of a sample of methylation percentages of the FOXA2 gene. In the histogram the number under each bar refers to the lower limit of the range

(Section 3.9, **step 4**) are another option when assumptions of normality are inappropriate.

3.5 General Linear Model/Logistic Regression

The linear model specified above assumed a normal distribution for the random variation. Sometimes the response variable will be binary; that is, it can take two possible values, which can be referred to as *no* and *yes*, or as 0 and 1. A normal assumption makes no sense here, and so we fit a model which has a binary outcome. The usual choice in that case is what is termed a logistic regression, which is the most common type of what are referred to as generalized linear models.

For a binary outcome, we model the probability of a "yes" outcome. This does not directly suit a linear formulation, and so we consider instead the odds, which is defined for probability p as $p/(1 - p)$, and we suppose that the logarithm of the odds is a linear function of the explanatory variables:

$$\log(p/(1 - p)) = \beta_1 X_1 + \beta_2 X_2 + \beta_3 X_3 + \cdots$$

We now have a model which is similar to the linear one we had for continuous variables, and most aspects of the interpretation and inference are the same. The β coefficients are more difficult to interpret than in the linear model because of the transformed scale. The most common way to present them is as odds ratios (OR), which are $\exp(\beta)$. They estimate the increase in odds associated with a unit increase in the explanatory X variable, or with membership of some group, relative to the reference group, in the case of categorical variables (*see* **Notes 8** and **9**).

3.6 Statistical Power

This is an issue which ideally is part of the design of a study, and is used to choose the number of observations to ensure that effects of a particular size will be detected if they should exist. Even if other constraints such as sample availability, time, and cost have determined the sample size, an awareness of the power can help with the interpretation of whatever results are found. We will discuss power in two contexts, that of estimation and of testing.

For estimation, we wish to present a population summary of some quantity, such as mean methylation of some gene, or the proportion of individuals in which it exceeds some specified value. For this we need to decide what standard error or confidence interval width we consider to be small enough. Standard error is $\sqrt{SD/n}$ or $\sqrt{p(1-p)/n}$. Confidence interval width is the standard error multiplied by t (the 95 % point of the t-distribution with degrees of freedom equal to the sample size, minus 1 for a mean, and which will always be close to 2).

Statistical power is a characteristic of hypothesis testing, where we examine data for evidence that a null hypothesis (usually absence of an effect or association) can be rejected. There are two types of incorrect conclusions in this situation: a false positive and false negative, traditionally known as type I and type II errors. The false positive rate is fixed by the choice of significance level. If it is 5 %, the most common choice, then there will be a 5 % false positive rate, and altering the experimental design or increasing the sample size will have no effect on this. The power is the converse of the false negative rate; that is, it is the probability that if an effect exists we will detect it by correctly rejecting the null hypothesis. This depends on the experimental design, sample size, and what the effect size in fact is—we are more likely to detect larger effects (*see* **Note 10**).

Power calculations can be approached in different ways. The power, the sample size, and detectable effect size are interrelated, and if any two are specified, the third may be calculated. The calculation is widely available in software and tables. The simplest situation is comparing two groups, in which case the formula for sample size is

$$n = 2(Z + T)^2 \sigma^2 / \delta^2$$

n is the sample size, σ is the standard deviation of variability within a group, and δ is the difference between groups that we wish to be able to detect. Z depends on the power of the test (it is the corresponding point of the standard normal distribution) and T depends on the significance level of the test. It also depends on n, so that the above equation needs to be solved rather than calculated, although we may approximate that $T = 2$, as long as the resulting value for n is no less than 15 (*see* **Note 11**).

3.7 High Dimensionality, Principal Components, and Other Multivariate Methods

The methods discussed in this section differ from all those covered earlier in that we no longer are developing a model for an outcome or response variable. We have a number of measurement variables, possibly very many, and are interested in exploring the patterns in their variability. We don't regard one of them as a response, but consider all on an equal basis. Nor are we aiming to test hypotheses

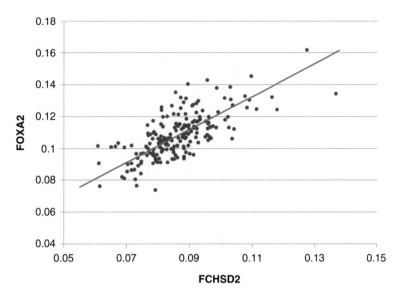

Fig. 2 Scatterplot of FOXA2 vs. FCHSD2 methylation, with first principal component axis

or validate models, so no p-values are produced. There are many multivariate methods, depending on the structure of the data and the patterns of interest. Here we present one of the most commonly used of these, PCA. The ideas on which it is based form the foundation of many other multivariate methods.

PCA can be viewed in a number of ways, but the usual one is as a way of reducing the dimensionality of a data set with many variables, which are usually correlated with each other. The idea is that although we may have recorded, say, 20 or 200 or 200,000 variables, there are not really that many dimensions of important interesting variability in the data. We suspect the variation of interest can be captured in fewer dimensions, and PCA aims to find these.

Figure 2 shows a scatterplot of just two methylation variables recorded in 192 subjects. Clearly these values are correlated. A line is shown fitted to the scatterplot. If we record where an observation is along this line (i.e., projected onto it), we will have captured most of the variability in two variables (FCHSD2 and FOXA2 methylation) in a single variable (position along the line). This is the first principal component.

Formally, it is the linear combination of the variables which maximizes the variability. It does not of course capture *all* of the variability. There is some variation perpendicular to the first component line. This perpendicular displacement is the second principal component. Formally, it is the linear combination perpendicular (and hence statistically uncorrelated) to the first which maximizes variability. And with two original variables, this is as far as we can go. Calculating these first two components can be seen as rotating the axes of the plot so that as much as possible of the variation is along the first axis. PCA generalizes this procedure to any number of variables. The maximum number of components is the number of original variables, or the number of observations minus one, if that is fewer. If we use all of these, we have not achieved a dimensionality reduction. The expectation is that the first few will contain most of the variation of interest. Reducing two variables to one, as we have done here, does not achieve much. But reducing 30 or 300,000 to 4, for example, would make discussing the patterns of variation much more tractable (*see* **Notes 12–14**).

3.8 Multiple Comparisons and False Discovery Rates

The traditional approach to statistical testing is to declare that sufficient evidence for an effect or association has been observed when the probability of as much evidence (as indicated by a difference or correlation or other statistic) occurring by chance is less than some value, usually 5 %. This implies that when tests are carried out in the absence of any effect or association 5 % of them will appear to be significant, wrongly implying an effect. These are termed false positives. As the number of tests increases, the probability of at least some of them being false positives increases. This is often seen as undesirable, and the solution proposed is to adjust the p-values from the tests, with the aim of ensuring that the probability of at least one false positive in the whole set of tests is no more than 5 %.

There are many ways of carrying out such adjustments, depending on how the set of tests which we wish to jointly "protect" from false positive risk is constructed. If the tests are all independent, then the Bonferroni correction can be used. If we are comparing a number of groups, then the comparisons are not independent, and Tukey's method is formulated for this situation. If the only comparisons of interest are for each group relative to a control, the Dunnett's test is appropriate (*see* **Note 15**).

Multiple comparison adjustment is not always desirable. In addition to the frequent difficulty of deciding which adjustment method is applicable, they all have the unavoidable effect of increasing the risk of false negatives; that is, where there are in fact effects or associations the adjusted test is more likely to declare them not to be significant. In some situations, the number of tests is large. This is generally the situation when methylation is recorded in arrays for example where a test at each site leads to a total of 10^5–10^6 tests in total. Attempting a multiple comparison adjustment in this situation will mean the loss of nearly all true effects as false negative risk approaches 100 %. What can help in this situation is to consider estimating the false positive rate from the data.

To see how this is done, first consider an experiment in which there is no treatment effect on any of the variables measured. In this case, any positive findings must be false. For each of the many variables, we will have calculated a p-value. The distribution of

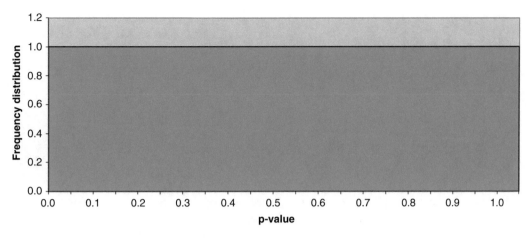

Fig. 3 Distribution of *p*-values when there are no effects

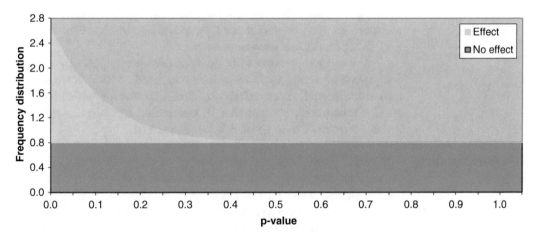

Fig. 4 Mixed distribution of *p*-values when there are some effects

these will be something like the plot below: they will be evenly spread between 0 and 1. 5 % of them will be less than $p = 0.05$ (Fig. 3).

Now suppose that we have an experiment where the treatments do have an effect on some of the variables. Let us suppose that 20 % of them are affected (although we do not know this in advance). For the 80 % which are unaffected, their *p*-values will be evenly spread between 0 and 1. For the 20 % which are affected, the *p*-values will have a distribution concentrated towards the lower end of the 0–1 range (Fig. 4).

By looking at the shape of this distribution, and possibly by fitting a mathematical curve to it, we can estimate how much of it is in the "no effect" (rectangular shaped) part, and how much is in "effect" part. Now suppose we choose a *p*-value cutoff in order to conclude which variables are affected. This will divide the variables

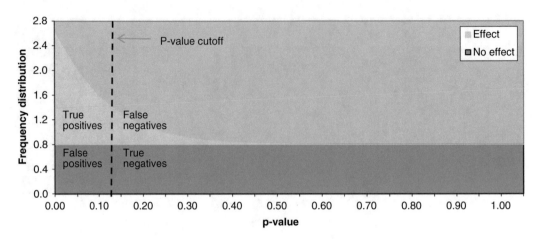

Fig. 5 Using a *p*-value cutoff to find significant effects

into four types. The *false discovery rate* is the proportion of variables chosen as positive which are false positives. In Fig. 5, it is about 50 % for the cutoff shown.

We can use it to quantify the false positive problem by estimating what percentage of the variables declared to be affected are not in fact affected. Alternatively, by choosing a value which we consider acceptable, we use that to determine the *p*-value cutoff to use—it doesn't have to be 5 % (*see* **Note 16**).

3.9 Other Statistical Methods

It is not possible in a single chapter to cover all of the statistical methods that might be relevant for studying methylation data. We have presented the most commonly used techniques, the linear model, logistic regression, and PCA. In this section we list some of the other methods that might be used, saying briefly what their purpose is, but without giving details.

1. *Mixed models*

The standard linear and logistic models accommodate only one source of random variation, usually between different subjects. Other sources of variation such as subject characteristics and treatments are considered "fixed" as they are what we are interested in studying and were not chosen at random. A mixed model allows two or more sources of random variation. This might be within subjects, or between centers in a multi-center study, where these were sampled from a larger population. Other possibilities are family, or pair in a twin or matched case–control study, and it can also be used for batch effects. The results of fitting a mixed model are similar to a standard linear model, with additional variance components estimated for each random effect. Significance tests for fixed effects are less straightforward however. Examples of the application of this approach to epigenetic analysis can be found in [15, 16].

2. *Repeated measures*

These are data where an outcome variable is recorded at multiple time points. Time is different from other factors in that it follows in a specific sequence and cannot be randomized. It is also usually the case that random variation at a time point is correlated with that at previous time points. Simple approaches involve looking at each time point separately, or calculating and modeling some summary of all time points. More sophisticated approaches model the pattern of change over time, and adapt to or model the correlation over time. Mixed models are a popular option in this case (*see* **Note 17**). Examples of the application of this approach to epigenetic analysis can be found in [8, 17].

3. *Survival data*

In some studies, the outcome of interest is death or survival of the subjects. This is not just a binary outcome, as the time until death is also of importance. The outcome recorded is this survival time, but the data are censored in that the survival time of some subjects is not known when the study is finished. The statistical analysis of such data is based on modeling the probability of survival as a function of time, and how this is affected by explanatory variables of interest. Examples of the application of this approach to epigenetic analysis can be found in [18, 19].

4. *Nonparametric methods*

These avoid assuming any particular distribution for the outcome variable, and so are an option when assumptions of normality of random variation, for example, are inappropriate, even after transformation. Typically they are based on using the rank rather than the absolute value of data observations. Versions for anything other than quite basic situations are difficult to find, and for smaller sample sizes they have less statistical power than tests based on a linear model. Examples of the application of this approach to epigenetic analysis can be found in [20, 21].

5. *The Bayesian philosophy*

The traditional view in statistics is that nature is fixed and data are variable, and so we make probability statements about data. The Bayesian view reverses this, and sees the data, once collected, as fixed, while our uncertainty about nature is best expressed using probability. This has advantages of logical consistency, but is more demanding to implement. It also requires that prior probabilities are stated, which of necessity are subjective, though these can often be made vague and uninformative. Examples of the application of this approach to epigenetic analysis can be found in [22–24].

3.10 Pathway Analysis

Most of the techniques above consider methylation values as abstract mathematical objects. However, their biological context can also be usefully included in the statistical analysis. The influences on and effects of methylation levels at different genome sites do not take place in isolation from other sites. A fuller picture is likely if we look at methylation in the context of patterns at related sites. One way to do this is by pathway analysis which utilizes the information within the sequence of genes in metabolic pathways. This involves looking at all the genes involved in a meaningful biochemical pathway such as glycolysis. Pathway analysis requires that we have data on methylation at many sites in the genome, such as is routinely provided in array-based methods.

A first step is to obtain pathway information from some suitable source. The Kyoto Encyclopaedia of Genes and Genomes (KEGG; http://www.genome.jp/kegg/pathway.html) [25] is a public pathway database resource, consisting of various pathway maps integrated from biological, chemical, molecular interaction and reaction networks of various organisms. It contains complete and well-organized metabolic pathways covering a wide range of organisms including human. Genes involved in a particular pathway or interconnected pathways are linked or interlinked by nodes, with different reference nodes annotated for different types of organisms. In general, pathways in *homo sapiens* are represented by reference node hsa:XXXX as the KEGG Pathway Identifiers (*see* **Note 18**).

It may be appropriate to standardize the methylation data by subtracting the mean methylation across all sites for each subject in order to focus on the pathway-specific effects. The analysis for a specific site depends on the nature of the study in question but the same analysis can be repeated for all sites that have been identified. The next step is to look for patterns in the summary statistics or in significance tests that have been calculated. The number of significant differences, possibly broken down by site categories (such as CpG or functional classification), may provide stronger evidence for an additional insight into the behavior of methylation variation in the pathway being examined. A pathway is not just a collection of genes, but it has a specific sequence and coherent blocks of change, and local clusters of positive or negative effects, that are generally more indicative of true biological significance than the usual approach of looking at the most statistically significant changes. This may be done using smoothing methods such as moving averages, kernel- and spline-based techniques, and locally weighted scatterplot smoothing (LOESS) [26] to reveal such local hotspots. These approaches can also be applied to the first-order differences as methylation effects may present as gradual changes between positive and negative effects. A global search in each pathway for evidence that the number of significant effects exceeds that expected by type I error rates can also be carried out. Autocorrelation between methylation in different genes can be estimated and used in calculating family-wise p-values. Another related approach is to carry out PCA on the methylation status of genes within specific pathways in order to identify the essential pathway epigenetic variance. In this analysis the estimated treatment effects and p-values obtained for the scores on the first components explain most of the variance [27–30].

4 Notes

1. One option is to randomize layout, allocating samples to batches completely randomly. Even better is some sort of restricted randomization involving blocking. This is a general principle in experimental design, and is discussed in more detail in [31, 32]. Instead of allocating samples randomly to batches, we aim for balance or try to have as many comparison of interest as possible within each batch. If there are a number of treatments for example, we try to have the same number of each treatment group in each batch, or the same number of each combination of the factors of interest.

2. A comparison of normalization methods was undertaken by [33], who found that they do not completely remove batch effects.

3. If looking at a sequential analysis of variance table (often termed "type 1 sums of squares") then batch should be included first in the sequence, as this will mean that any confounding with batch effects will not affect subsequent terms. If such confounding has been avoided by design, then the order should be unimportant.

4. Thus the coefficients denote the difference between that group and the reference group. If there are n groups, then there will be $n - 1$ coefficients to represent the grouping variable.

5. There is a disadvantage to turning a continuous variable into categories, and that is the loss of information it implies. The usual BMI categories, for example, imply no difference between two individuals with BMIs of 25.5 and 29.5, while the latter is in a different category from someone with a BMI of 30.5. There is also a loss of statistical power if the analysis does not account for the ordering of the categories, which very often it does not. In terms of variance information discarded, defining tertiles discards about 21 % of the variability, quartiles discards about 14 %, and quintiles discards about 10 %.

6. Normality can be assessed by inspecting the form of the distribution or by formal tests. No data will be exactly normally distributed, and so will always fail the tests if the sample size is

large enough, even if the departures from normality are not enough to be a problem. But such tests can be useful if an objective procedure is required.

7. Log transforms are the most common type, and change multiplicative differences into additive ones (i.e., two pairs of numbers with the same ratio, such as 2 and 4 and 7 and 14, will have the same difference after a log transform). Logs will only change the shape of a distribution substantially if the ratio between the highest and lowest values is more than 2 or 3. The base chosen for logs (10, e, 2) only has a constant scaling effect of the numbers, like choosing between cm and mm for length.

8. An advantage of odds ratios is that it can be shown that estimates from a case–control study, although an artificial construction, are valid estimates for the whole population.

9. The odds scale for risk is not as clear as the original probability scale, and so other methods which more directly model the probabilities, such as Poisson regression, can be used [34]. These will produce effect estimates on other scales, such as relative risk, which is simply a ratio of probabilities.

10. The effect size to use in a calculation might be the effect size you expect, if you are confident of this, but arguably it should be the smallest effect size you would not want to miss. Where this is difficult to specify, it is possible to use effect sizes expressed relative to the natural random variability. For comparing two groups, Cohen's D is defined as the difference in means relative to the standard deviation within groups. Effects are termed small, medium, and large for values of 0.2, 0.5, and 1.0.

11. Many statistical programs and websites offer a power and sample size calculations for a wide variety of situations

12. One point to note is that the line in Fig. 2 is *not* the regression line. The first principal component is symmetric with respect to the two variables, whereas linear regression is not: it treats one variable as explanatory and the other as the response. The resulting fitted lines are different.

13. Standardizing the variables as part of PCA is a common choice. This means scaling them all to have the same variance (standard deviation) so that those which are numerically more variable do not thereby contribute more to the calculation of components. It is the usual choice when the variables being examined have different units. If the variables do in fact all have the same units, as will be the case if all are methylation percentages, then not standardizing should be considered, if those variables with greater variability are more important because of this. Standardizing or not is often expressed as basing the PCA on the

correlation or covariance matrix, respectively, or in scaling or not the original variables.

14. With PCA, it is often examination of plots of the component scores which is most useful. Thought should be given to including more information in these plots, such as by coloring the points, or using different symbols, according to whatever groupings are present in the observations. If there appears to be difference in the point scatter according to these groups, it indicates that overall they are a source of variability in the set of variables.

15. The option of doing no multiple comparison adjustment should also be considered. Such adjustments have a highly undesirable effect on false negative error rates. Simply omitting them and leaving it to the reader to bear in mind that a scattering of significant p-values will occur by chance may be a more suitable approach for exploratory studies, rather than those intended to rigorously test hypotheses. Where many results are presented, it is the overall pattern, frequency, and strength of the significant results which tell a story.

16. It may well be asked at this point that having quantified the false positives, can we not say which ones they are? Unfortunately this cannot be done. The only way to find out is to do some more research. To be fully valid, this further research needs to be carried out on new biological samples, and not by some other technology with the original samples.

17. This mixed model approach to repeated measures is considered "state of the art" at present. Care is needed in choosing and specifying these models, particularly regarding the form of autocorrelation between time points. *Autoregressive* models assume that current values are influenced by only the most recent past values, *moving-average* models assume that random influences are smoothed over time, and *antedependence* models are suitable for time points which are not uniformly spaced.

18. KEGG itself has limited gene name conversion ability and other resources such as the Hyperlink Management System (HMS) systems (http://biodb.jp/) can be used to link KEGG names to, for example, Illumina index file gene names.

Acknowledgement

This work was supported by the Scottish Government's Rural and Environment Science and Analytical Services Division.

References

1. Wu HC, Wang Q, Yang HI, Tsai WY, Chen CJ, Santella RM (2012) Global DNA methylation levels in white blood cells as a biomarker for hepatocellular carcinoma risk: a nested case-control study. Carcinogenesis 33 (7):1340–1345

2. Canivell S, Ruano EG, Sisó-Almirall A, Kostov B, González-de Paz L, Fernandez-Rebollo E, Hanzu F, Párrizas M, Novials A, Gomis R (2013) Gastric inhibitory polypeptide receptor methylation in newly diagnosed, drug-naïve patients with type 2 diabetes: a case-control study. PLoS One 8(9):e75474

3. Kuchiba A, Iwasaki M, Ono H, Kasuga Y, Yokoyama S, Onuma H, Nishimura H, Kusama R, Tsugane S, Yoshida T (2014) Global methylation levels in peripheral blood leukocyte DNA by LUMA and breast cancer: a case-control study in Japanese women. Br J Cancer 110(11):2765–2771

4. Su S, Zhu H, Xu X, Wang X, Dong Y, Kapuku G, Treiber F, Gutin B, Harshfield G, Snieder H, Wang X (2014) DNA methylation of the LY86 gene is associated with obesity, insulin resistance, and inflammation. Twin Res Hum Genet 17(3):183–191

5. King WD, Ashbury JE, Taylor SA, Tse MY, Pang SC, Louw JA, Vanner SJ (2014) A cross-sectional study of global DNA methylation and risk of colorectal adenoma. BMC Cancer 14:488

6. Voisin S, Almén MS, Moschonis G, Chrousos GP, Manios Y, Schiöth HB (2015) Dietary fat quality impacts genome-wide DNA methylation patterns in a cross-sectional study of Greek preadolescents. Eur J Hum Genet 23 (5):654–662

7. Cecil CA, Lysenko LJ, Jaffee SR, Pingault JB, Smith RG, Relton CL, Woodward G, McArdle W, Mill J, Barker ED (2014) Environmental risk, Oxytocin Receptor Gene (OXTR) methylation and youth callous-unemotional traits: a 13-year longitudinal study. Mol Psychiatry 9 (10):1071–1077

8. Simpkin AJ, Suderman M, Gaunt TR, Lyttleton O, McArdle WL, Ring SM, Tilling K, Davey Smith G, Relton CL (2015) Longitudinal analysis of DNA methylation associated with birth weight and gestational age. Hum Mol Genet 24(13):3752–3763

9. Feinberg JI, Bakulski KM, Jaffe AE, Tryggvadottir R, Brown SC, Goldman LR, Croen LA, Hertz-Picciotto I, Newschaffer CJ, Daniele Fallin M, Feinberg AP (2015) Paternal sperm DNA methylation associated with early signs of autism risk in an autism-enriched cohort. Int J Epidemiol 44:1199

10. Bollati V, Schwartz J, Wright R, Litonjua A, Tarantini L, Suh H, Sparrow D, Vokonas P, Baccarelli A (2009) Decline in genomic DNA methylation through aging in a cohort of elderly subjects. Mech Ageing Dev 30 (4):234–239

11. Briollais L, Ozcelik H, Kwiatkowski M, Xu J, Savas S, Olkhov E, Recker F, Kuk C, Hanna S, Fleshner NE, Juvet T, Friedlander M, Li H, Chadwick K, Trachtenberg J, Toi A, Van Der Kwast TH, Diamandis EP, Bapat B, Zlotta AR (2015) Functional role of the kallikrein 6 region of the kallikrein locus in genetic predisposition for aggressive (Gleason ≥8) prostate cancer: fine-mapping and methylation study in a Canadian cohort and the Swiss arm of the European Randomized Study for Prostate Cancer Screening. J Urol Suppl 14(2):e42

12. Yousefi P, Huen K, Schall RA, Decker A, Elboudwarej E, Quach H, Barcellos L, Holland N (2013) Considerations for normalization of DNA methylation data by Illumina 450K BeadChip assay in population studies. Epigenetics 8(11):1141–1152

13. Khan A, Rayner GD (2003) Robustness to non-normality of common tests for the many-sample location problem. J Appl Math Decis Sci 7:187–206

14. Beasley TM, Erickson S, Allison DB (2009) Rank-based inverse normal transformations are increasingly used, but are they merited? Behav Genet 39:580–595

15. Hou L, Zhang X, Tarantini L, Nordio F, Bonzini M, Angelici L, Marinelli B, Rizzo G, Cantone L, Apostoli P, Bertazzi PA, Baccarelli A (2011) Ambient PM exposure and DNA methylation in tumor suppressor genes: a cross-sectional study. Part Fibre Toxicol 8:25. doi:10.1186/1743-8977-8-25

16. Smith AK, Conneely KN, Newport DJ, Kilaru V, Schroeder JW, Pennell PB, Knight BT, Cubells JC, Stowe ZN, Brennan PA (2012) Prenatal antiepileptic exposure associates with neonatal DNA methylation differences. Epigenetics 7(5):458–463. doi:10.4161/epi.19617

17. Rusiecki JA, Byrne C, Galdzicki Z, Srikantan V, Chen L, Poulin M, Yan L, Baccarelli A (2013) PTSD and DNA methylation in select immune function gene promoter regions: a repeated measures case-control study of U.S. military service members. Front Psychiatry 4:56

18. Inamura K, Yamauchi M, Nishihara R, Lochhead P, Qian ZR, Kuchiba A, Kim SA, Mima K,

Sukawa Y, Jung S, Zhang X, Wu K, Cho E, Chan AT, Meyerhardt JA, Harris CC, Fuchs CS, Ogino S (2014) Tumor LINE-1 methylation level and microsatellite instability in relation to colorectal cancer prognosis. J Natl Cancer Inst 106(9): pii: dju195. doi: 10.1093/jnci/dju195

19. Shigeyasu K, Nagasaka T, Mori Y, Yokomichi N, Kawai T, Fuji T, Kimura K, Umeda Y, Kagawa S, Goel A, Fujiwara T (2015) Clinical significance of MLH1 methylation and CpG island methylator phenotype as prognostic markers in patients with gastric cancer. PLoS One 10(6):e0130409. doi:10.1371/journal.pone.0130409

20. de Arruda IT, Persuhn DC, de Oliveira NF (2013) The MTHFR C677T polymorphism and global DNA methylation in oral epithelial cells. Genet Mol Biol 36(4):490–493

21. Mirabello L, Schiffman M, Ghosh A, Rodriguez AC, Vasiljevic N, Wentzensen N, Herrero R, Hildesheim A, Wacholder S, Scibior-Bentkowska D, Burk RD, Lorincz AT (2013) Elevated methylation of HPV16 DNA is associated with the development of high grade cervical intraepithelial neoplasia. Int J Cancer 132 (6):1412–1422

22. Melnikov A, Scholtens D, Godwin A, Levenson V (2009) Differential methylation profile of ovarian cancer in tissues and plasma. J Mol Diagn 11(1):60–65

23. Beggs AD, Jones A, El-Bahrawy M, Abulafi M, Hodgson SV, Tomlinson IP (2013) Whole-genome methylation analysis of benign and malignant colorectal tumours. J Pathol 229 (5):697–704

24. Bonello N, Sampson J, Burn J, Wilson IJ, McGrown G, Margison GP, Thorncroft M, Crossbie P, Povey AC, Santibanez-Koref M, Walters K (2013) Bayesian inference supports a location and neighbour-dependent model of DNA methylation propagation at the MGMT gene promoter in lung tumours. J Theor Biol 336:87–95

25. Kanehisa M, Goto S (2000) KEGG: kyoto encyclopedia of genes and genomes. Nucleic Acids Res 28(1):27–30

26. Cleveland WS, Devlin SJ (1988) Locally-weighted regression: an approach to regression analysis by local fitting. J Am Stat Assoc 83:596–610

27. Yang L, Tong ML, Chi X, Zhang M, Zhang CM, Guo XR (2012) Genomic DNA methylation changes in NYGGF4-overexpression 3T3-L1 adipocytes. Int J Mol Sci 13(12):15575–15587

28. Li B, Lu Q, Song ZG, Yang L, Jin H, Li ZG, Zhao TJ, Bai YF, Zhu J, Chen HZ, Xu ZY (2013) Functional analysis of DNA methylation in lung cancer. Eur Rev Med Pharmacol Sci 17(9):1191–1197

29. Finer S, Mathews C, Lowe R, Smart M, Hillman S, Foo L, Sinha A, Williams D, Rakyan VK, Hitman GA (2015) Maternal gestational diabetes is associated with genome-wide DNA methylation variation in placenta and cord blood of exposed offspring. Hum Mol Genet 24(11):3021–3029

30. del Rosario MC, Ossowski V, Knowler WC, Bogardus C, Baier LJ, Hanson RL (2014) Potential epigenetic dysregulation of genes associated with MODY and type 2 diabetes in humans exposed to a diabetic intrauterine environment: an analysis of genome-wide DNA methylation. Metabolism 63(5):654–660

31. Addelman S (1969) The generalized randomized block design. Am Stat 23(4):35–36. doi:10.2307/2681737

32. Bailey RA (2008) Design of comparative experiments. Cambridge University Press, Cambridge. ISBN 978-0-521-68357-9

33. Sun Z, Chai HS, Wu Y, White WM, Donkena KV, Klein CJ, Garovic VD, Therneau TM, Kocher JP (2011) Batch effect correction for genome-wide methylation data with Illumina Infinium platform. BMC Med Genomics 4:84

34. Cameron AC, Trivedi PK (1998) Regression analysis of count data. Cambridge University Press, Cambridge. ISBN 0-521-63201-3

Methods in Molecular Biology (2017) 1589: 205–206
DOI 10.1007/978-1-4939-6903-6
© Springer Science+Business Media New York 2017

INDEX

Printed in the United States
By Bookmasters